Activities
and
the "Well Elderly"

Activities
and
the "Well Elderly"

Phyllis M. Foster
Editor

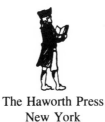

The Haworth Press
New York

Activities and the "Well Elderly" has also been published as *Activities, Adaptation & Aging,* Volume 3, Number 2, Winter 1982.

The Haworth Press, Inc. 28 East 22 Street, New York, NY 10010

Library of Congress Cataloging in Publication Data
Main entry under title:

Activities and the "well elderly."

"Has also been published as Activities, adaptation & aging, volume 3, number 2, winter 1982."
 Includes bibliographies and index.
 1. Aged—Addresses, essays, lectures. 2. Aged—United States—Addresses, essays, lectures. I. Foster, Phyllis M.
HQ1061.A29   1983   305.2'6   83-4326
ISBN 0-86656-230-3

Activities and the "Well Elderly"

Activities, Adaptation & Aging
Volume 3, Number 2

CONTENTS

From the Editor

It is with great pleasure that this special issue is presented to you, our readers! There is a tendency to think of all older people as living in some type of institutional setting; a fact that is simply not true! Those of us in the field of Gerontology know the reality of the situation to be that the majority of persons over the age of 65 actually remain in the community, continuing their life-long patterns of coping with life and living. How and why, are questions for which we continue to seek answers.

We do not mean to imply that this issue is the end-all, be-all to what is happening in communities with the well elderly. Much research, planning, and programming continues; some will be found within these pages. It is our desire that after perusing what is presented here, you will want to share the results of your findings and what you are doing, so that another special issue evolves.

We dedicate this particular issue to the "Well Elderly," as we explore a variety of their activities, adaptations and aging.

P.M.F.

Old Versus Aging

Phyllis M. Foster

"Old" is a state of mind that is largely dependent upon how one feels about oneself at any particular point in time and depends a great deal on mental attitude. Each of us has our own definition of "old," and that is generally about ten years from our own age! As we get older, that span continues to stay some distance from our own age. The social and cultural environments in which one has been raised also contribute to one's attitude toward "old." Old "things" increase in value and are treasured as antiques. Old people however, are thought to be weak, dependent, senile, talkative, out of touch and close-minded! There seems to be a prejudice in our society towards aging and the aged. Unfortunately, the victims of that prejudice tend to believe those negative definitions of themselves and may very well accept and even expect the treatment they receive.

"Aging," on the other hand, is a normal part of the development of the human being that, like any other stage of development, produces particular needs and stresses. Depending upon the social and

Phyllis Foster is currently a Therapeutic Activities Consultant to Long Term Care Facilities, in private practice, and Editor of this journal. She is also involved in providing pre-retirement classes and facilitating support groups on "Aging with your Aging Parents" for a number of churches. Mrs. Foster has worked in the field of activities management with the aged for 19 years, both in long term care facilities and in a hospital-based geriatric clinic. In 1978, she was the recipient of the American Health Care Association's Better Life Award, Humanitarian Services for Outstanding Achievement in Caring for the Needs of the Elderly. Most recently, she was awarded the 1982 Vesta Bowden Award, from the Colorado Health Care Association, for her contributions to the health care profession through education. Mrs. Foster is listed in the "Who's Who of American Women," 1981 and 1982.

cultural environments in which one lives, as well as the capabilities and disabilities one possesses, the changes which occur in all life stages are always very individual.

An individual consists of many facets which identify him, the most conspicuous of these being his name. When carried in the womb, much discussion prevails concerning a name; when born in a hospital, the infant is identified with a "name bracelet"; the first thing people want to know is, "what did you name him?" All through life the individual carries that name as a means of identification, and in death the name is transcribed on a tombstone to identify one to posterity. All people begin to establish their identity with a name; who we are!

Physical appearance further identifies an individual: big/small; fat/thin; hair; features; facial expressions; attractive or not. That identity is then broadened even more by relationships with others, preferred activities, the things that are of importance to the individual, the roles experienced in a lifetime and their significance. Family roles and relationships involved in being a child, sibling, adult, spouse, parent, and/or grandparent, as well as the roles and interaction experienced in church, clubs, schools, friendships, and especially the work role, all demonstrate an individual's value to society. The identity is further expanded by one's life experiences; what the individual has done with his life and what life has done to him; how he meets his other needs, such as dealing with frustrations, achievements and failures, likes and dislikes, hopes and fears; what his capabilities are and what expectations he has, or once had. These, one's life experiences, complete each person as a unique individual; what and why we are!

Throughout life development, that unique individual attempts to hold fast to his identity, but nowhere is this as evident as in the maturing years. Generally the name is retained, although sometimes altered to "Grandpa," "the old man," or "Pops." Gradual physical changes which have negative connotations appear: the hair gradually grays; wrinkles and/or age spots emerge; glasses, dentures, and/or hearing aids may be needed; and the capacity for physical activity may become more limited. Roles will have changed many times, losing some and gaining others through the years, but if over 65, the very significant work role may be lost and the individual is now called "retired" and must learn to live on a fixed income. Younger people have supplanted him in his former roles. Relationships with spouse, family and friends may have disappeared through death and/or separation and the individual begins to confront the inevitability of his own demise; he stands alone.

These changes are commonly termed "losses": physical losses, social losses, and economic losses. These losses in later life are a direct cause of loneliness in which the older person will expend enormous amounts of physical and emotional energy in grieving and resolving that grief, in adapting to changes that result from the losses, and in recovering from the stresses inherent in these processes. No matter what the loss, its absence will create a gap in life's continuity. That unique individual, that vital human being, may very well succumb to a crumbled self-concept and self-esteem; or, he may "roll with the punches" and come up fighting. . . fighting to retain his identity as a contributing member of a society that gives all outward appearances of wanting to push him out! Ultimately the aging process produces biological/physical stresses that require assistance from others at a time when social/emotional resources are at their lowest and when economic assets are also diminished.

While this may seem to be a dismal view of getting older, this is not necessarily universal! In our lifetimes, mostly through trial and error, we do discover what works and what doesn't work for us as we learn to cope with stress. That learning stays with us throughout our lives; although we all need support from time to time in coping with that stress. Fortunately, we are finding increased community support systems that are geared to assisting older people in staying in their own homes and environments, for as long as possible.

While the process of aging creates specific needs for the elderly, gerontology professionals must accept the challenge of helping to meet those needs. We do this through providing good physical care, overseeing proper nutrition, providing meaningful activities, encouraging social contacts with peers, developing a feeling of usefulness, and supporting the highest level of wellness and independence possible. We must have expectations of our clients while allowing them opportunities to take risks. Life and living is a risk! In this way, the older people we work with will be assisted in regaining and/or maintaining feelings of dignity, self-worth, and their uniqueness as an individual.

ETCHINGS

Ride My Umbrella

Elizabeth Williams

Shattered by the wind, the liquid jewels
Of heaven tear against my window pane.
There's terror that my logic ridicules
In every vein. I'm humbled by such rain.
What signs I know I make against mad ghouls
That howl in faceless pleasure at my pain.

By seven locks I'm sealed apart. I hide
Inside this house that once knew open doors.
No longer have I friends to match my stride.
It's not the same. Fierce water moats my shores.
Once linked, I'm now an island 'gainst the tide
That all but I—inside—seem to ignore.

The hairy skies deny my need to go
Beyond this shrinking world. It's not my fault!
I lived too long—and live I shall! I know,
By my umbrella vague attacks can halt.
I'll risk that skill, not like Lot's wife, let grow
The others while I stay and turn to salt.

Written to an old woman, alone in Manhattan who K.O.'d a purse-snatcher with her umbrella and refused to move or stay inside her apartment.

Elizabeth Williams began her writing career in Europe during the 1960s, publishing poems and short stories in women's and small magazines. Produced as a playwright in the 1970s, she continues to publish, turning her attention to non-fiction as well and looking at the very young and fairly old, for inspiration.

Correlates of Loneliness
among the Black Elderly

Robert F. Creecy
Roosevelt Wright
William E. Berg

ABSTRACT. The purpose of this study was to examine the relationship of selected demographic, activity and social-psychological variables to feelings of loneliness among a national sample of non-institutionalized black elderly. Findings indicated that only the activity and social-psychological variables had significant relationship with feelings of loneliness. Implications of the findings for intervention are discussed.

Loneliness is a universal human phenomenon and there is probably no one who has not felt lonely at some time. While current estimates of the prevalence of loneliness in the general population are unavailable, there is evidence that it may be rather widespread among the elderly. The results of a recent national survey suggest that approximately 12% of the elderly population, or some 2.6 million persons age 65 and over, view loneliness as a major personal problem (Harris & Associates, 1975).

Weiss (1973) describes loneliness as an uncanny feeling that is uniformly distressing. Although it has been suggested feelings of loneliness among the elderly are intrinsically connected with enduring social isolation (Gordon, 1975), there is not unanimous support for this view. Polcino (1978), for example, observes that some individuals may feel loneliness in the midst of a group of people and

Robert F. Creecy, PhD, is Associate Professor, College of Social Work, University of South Carolina, Columbia, SC 29208. Roosevelt Wright, PhD is Assistant Professor, Graduate School of Social Work, University of Texas at Arlington, Arlington, TX 76019. William E. Berg, PhD is Associate Professor, School of Social Welfare, University of Wisconsin, Milwaukee, WI 53201.

9

others who experience only minimal levels of social exchange may not feel lonely at all. Hoskisson (1963) notes that:

> Loneliness is a *conscious* experience of separation from something or someone desired, required or needed. It is not solitariness, for there the separation may not be felt, nor is it lack of physical or social contact, for as we know the presence of people does not necessarily assuage it. So there must be experienced a need, a desire for contact, and an inability to make it.

Loneliness is a painful, frightening experience and has detrimental effects on the general well-being of the elderly. In fact, practitioners such as Fromm-Reichman (1959) report that persons tend to suppress memory of earlier experiences of loneliness because recall of these experiences would be threatening to their current well-being. When facing prolonged and severe loneliness, in the words of one observer, "elderly persons are frequently unable to sleep, may lose the will to eat, and eventually the will to live" (Hawkins, 1978).

Previous research has identified a number of factors which are associated with feelings of loneliness in old age (Atchley, 1977; Berg et al., 1981; Bond, 1954; Dean, 1962; Kivett, 1979; Shanas et al., 1968; Townsend, 1973; Woodward et al., 1974). Virtually all of the studies in this area, however, are based on white populations. As a consequence, factors which are associated with feelings of loneliness among black elderly have, for the most part, remained uninvestigated.

To partially rectify this situation, the present study focused on a sample of older black adults. The purpose of the study was to examine and assess correlates of loneliness among this population subgroup.

STUDY DESIGN

The data used in this study were drawn from a national survey of the non-institutionalized adult population of the United States. Conducted by Louis Harris and Associates, the survey was designed to gather information on the public's perception of aging and to obtain data on the attitudes and conditions of the elderly. The stratified multistage cluster sample was comprised of 4,254 individuals who were interviewed during the spring and summer of 1974. The present study uses only data from the 479 black elderly (11% of the total sample) included in the broader survey.

Respondents were between fifty-five and ninety-four years of age with a mean age of 65.3 years. Females comprised 54% of the sample and 46% were male. As might be expected for an older black population, the respondents' educational levels were quite low; 95% had a high school education or less. The median household income was $4,321. Over half (53%) of the group was married, 28% were widowed and the remaining 19% were either separated, divorced or never married. Their average number of children was 2.9. Nearly half (49%) of the respondents lived in rural areas; most of the rest were central city residents (39%).

Feelings of loneliness, the dependent or criterion variable in this analysis, was determined via the question "would you say that loneliness is hardly a problem, a somewhat serious problem, or a very serious problem for you?" The coded responses ranged from 1 for "hardly a problem" to 3 for "a very serious problem."

Fourteen independent variables were included in this study. These variables were grouped into three conceptual categories: demographic, activity and social-psychological.

The demographic category included age, sex and marital status. The age of each respondent was coded as actual age; sex was coded as a dummy variable with a score of 0 for males and 1 for females; marital status was also treated as a dummy variable with 0 indicating non-married and 1 coded as married.

There are six activity variables. The first is a 20-point index which is a measure of the amount of contact the respondent had with relatives and close friends. The final five—time spent working, time spent reading, time spent watching television, time spent with hobbies and participating in clubs, fraternal or community organizations—were all based on responses to the question, "Do you spend hardly any time, some but not a lot, or a lot of time participating in these activities?" The coded responses ranged from 1 for "hardly any time" to 3 for a "a lot of time."

The final category, social-psychological, included five variables—fear of crime, not enough friends, not feeling needed, poor health and financial inadequacy. Each of these variables was measured by asking, "Would you say that these areas are not a problem, a somewhat serious problem, or a very serious problem for you?" The responses were coded 1, 2 and 3, respectively.

Pearsonian correlation coefficients were computed to determine the nature of the relationships between the independent variables and the dependent variable, feelings of loneliness. The present level of statistical significance for this study was .05.

FINDINGS AND DISCUSSION

A review of the data presented in Table 1 reveals that nine of the fourteen independent variables have significant relationships with loneliness. Of the three categories of variables, only one does not statistically relate. All of the demographic variables have only negligible relationships with loneliness within this study population.

Inspection of the activity category indicates that significant relationships exist between four of the six independent variables and the dependent variable. Feelings of loneliness are associated with decreased contact with relatives and close friends, a low degree of reading and spending limited time working. On the other hand, spending a great deal of time viewing television is associated with higher levels of loneliness. With regard to the social-psychological variables, each has a significant relationship with the dependent variable. The fact that these relationships are positive suggest that black elderly who tend to consider fear of crime, not enough friends, not feeling needed, poor health and inadequate finances as serious personal problems also tend to feel lonely.

Some of the above findings are inconsistent with previous research on white populations. Studies by Shanas et al. (1968) and Berg et al. (1981) found, unlike the present investigation, sex to be a significant correlate of loneliness. Moreover, the finding of a lack of significance in the relationship between age and loneliness contrast markedly with Dean's (1962) data which indicate that feelings of loneliness vary directly with age. While the data reported here suggest that marital status has little effect on loneliness, others have observed that feelings of loneliness are differentiated on the basis of marital status (Lopata, 1973; Townsend, 1957), with the single (especially the widowed and divorced) having a rather strong propensity toward loneliness (Bond, 1954).

Barh and Harvey's (1979) contention that contact with relatives and friends and viewing television have little impact on loneliness is not corroborated by our data. Findings from this study clearly suggest that frequent contact with family and friends relieves loneliness and the leisure activity of watching television, contrary to popular

Table 1: Correlations Between Independent Variables And Feelings of Loneliness Among the Black Elderly

Independent Variables	Correlation with Loneliness (N=479)
Demographic	
Age	.11
Sex	-.08
Marital Status	-.14
Activity	
Contact with Relatives and Close Friends	-.19*
Time Spent Working	-.25*
Time Spent Reading	-.17*
Time Spent Watching TV	.23**
Time Spent with Hobbies	-.06
Organizational Participation	.03
Social-Psychological	
Fear of Crime	.30***
Not Enough Friends	.50***
Not Feeling Needed	.54***
Perceived Health Problems	.51***
Perceived Financial Inadequacy	.41***

*	$p < .05$
**	$p < .01$
***	$p < .001$

belief, reinforces loneliness. Supportive of previous research, however, is the finding that activities such as working and reading act as antidotes to loneliness (Blau, 1973; Berg et al., 1981).

Self-evaluation of poor health and perceived financial inadequacy are, as this study indicates, closely associated with feelings of loneliness. These findings, which are consistent with prior research (Barh & Harvey, 1979; Shanas et al., 1968), are apparently implying that persons who regard themselves as lacking the resources of good health and financial solvency tend to live less than full and satisfying lives. Although the relationship of fear of crime to loneliness has not been examined in prior research, evidence offered by Lawton et al. (1977) lends credence to our finding of a significant relationship between these variables. These investigators report that this fear forces the elderly to curtail their usual activity patterns and lead a restricted and solitary existence.

The finding of a direct relationship between the variable not feeling needed and feelings of loneliness is in line with current theorizing about loneliness. According to Williams (1978), persons who feel unwanted or not needed by others find it difficult to make friendly overtures and establish interpersonal relationships. The inability to form desired relationships has been regarded as a primary cause of loneliness (Weiss, 1973). Indeed, the findings of this study reveal that persons who report not having enough friends are inclined to feel lonely.

SUMMARY AND IMPLICATIONS

In this study, correlates of loneliness among a national sample of noninstitutionalized black elderly were examined and assessed. While each of the demographic variables employed in this analysis has a very weak relationship with loneliness, most of the activity variables and all of the social-psychological variables are significantly associated with feelings of loneliness. These results have implications for loneliness intervention among black older people.

Participation in leisure activities and social groups which are entertaining or which link older persons with the outside community is widely heralded as an important remedy for loneliness (Burnside, 1971; Butler, 1975). Data from the present study indicate, however, that participation in only some of the activities and groups which have been designated as meeting these specifications is likely to be effective. The evidence suggests that integration into friendship groups, increased contact with friends and relatives, working and reading may offset feelings of loneliness; whereas organizational participation, involvement with hobbies and watching television may not counteract feelings of loneliness. As previously noted, those individuals who report viewing television on a frequent basis are actually more apt to experience loneliness than those who report limited exposure to this medium. Program planners and practitioners who are interested in loneliness intervention should be cognizant of the fact that activity in general may not be a satisfactory prescription for addressing the problem of loneliness among the black elderly.

The findings of this study indicate that perceived poor health and perceived financial inadequacy are directly linked to feelings of loneliness. Negative assessments of health and personal income tend to reduce mobility and prevent the black elderly from venturing beyond their residential contexts to participate in activities and social groups that may thwart feelings of loneliness. Health care services, both preventive and rehabilitative, should be implemented to address the health needs and requirements of black older people. Special provisions such as reduced fares for public transportation would be very helpful to those individuals who have limited incomes. The implementation of these measures may increase the mobility of older black adults and influence their predisposition to seek out and capitalize on social opportunities in the broader community arena.

Fear of crime, as do poor health and inadequate finances, leads to involuntary social isolation which in turn gives rise to feelings of loneliness. The implementation of security escort services and the installation of crime prevention devices such as mercury vapor lights may help minimize this fear and provide the elderly with increased opportunities for social interaction. These suggestions, of course, are far from new. Some municipalities have made concerted efforts to prevent crime and establish security services for the elderly. Practitioners who work with the aging should encourage policymakers to improve upon and extend these efforts to the neighborhoods and communities where the black elderly live.

Although the present study has identified several correlates of loneliness, much more empirical information is needed to devise a comprehensive plan for intervention. Future investigations should build on this study by examining the relationship of the entire range of demographic, activity and social-psychological variables to feelings of loneliness among the black elderly. Attention should be paid to the primary causes of loneliness; its long-term consequences and current interventive techniques should be evaluated. In addition to focusing on black elderly residents of the conventional community, these investigations should draw their samples from among black elderly who reside in the various institutional settings. The results of these efforts would enhance our understanding of loneliness and assist in developing a broad-based strategy for loneliness intervention within the black elderly population.

REFERENCES

Atchley, R. C. The social forces in later life (2nd ed.). Belmont, CA: Wadsworth, 1977.

Barh, H. M., & Harvey, C. D. Correlates of loneliness among widows bereaved in a mining disaster. *Psychological Reports*, 1979, *44*, 367-385.

Berg, S., Mellstrom, D., Persson, G., & Svanborg, A. Loneliness in the swedish aged. *Journal of Gerontology*, 1981, *36*, 342-349.

Blau, Z. S. *Old age in a changing society*. New York: New Viewpoint, 1973.

Bond, F., Barber, R. E., Vieg, J. A. Perry, L. B., Scaff, A. H. & Lee, L. J. *Our needy aged*. New York: Henry Holt & Co., 1954.

Burnside, I. M. Loneliness in old age. *Mental Hygiene*, 1971, *55*, 391-397.

Butler, R. *Why survive? Being old in America* (1st ed.). New York: Harper & Row, 1975.

Dean, L. R. Aging and the decline of affect. *Journal of Gerontology*, 1962, *17*, 440-446.

Fromm-Reichman, F. Loneliness. *Psychiatry*, 1959, *22*, 1-12.

Gordon, S. *Lonely in America*. New York: Simon & Schuster, 1976.

Harris, L., & Associates. *The myth and realities of aging in America*. The National Council on the Aging, Inc., Washington, D.C., 1975.

Hawkins, B. Mental health of the black aged. In L. E. Gary (Ed.), *Mental health: A challenge to the black community*. Philadelphia: Dorrance & Co., 1978.

Hoskisson, J. B. *Loneliness: An explanation, a cure*. New York: Citadel Press, 1963.

Kivett, V. R. Discriminators of loneliness among the rural elderly: Implications for intervention. *Gerontologist*, 1979, *19*, 108-115.

Lawton, M. P., Nahemo, L. Yaffee, S., & Feldman, S. Psychological aspects of crime and fear of crime. In J. Goldsmith & S. S. Goldsmith (Eds.), *Crime and elderly*. Lexington, MA: D.C. Heath, 1977.

Lopata, H. Z. Loneliness: Forms and components. *Social Problems*. 1968, *17*, 248-261.

Polcino, A. Loneliness—The genesis of solitude, friendship, and contemplation. *Hospital Progress*, 1979, *60*, 61-65.

Shanas, E., Townsend, P., Wedderburn, D., Friss, H., Milhoj, P., & Stehouwer, J. *Old people in three industrialized societies*. New York: Atherton, 1968.

Townsend, P. *The family life of old people*. London: Routledge & Kegan Paul, 1957.

_____. Isolation and loneliness in the aged. In R. S. Weiss (ed.), *Loneliness: The experience of emotional and social isolation*. MIT, Cambridge, MA, 1973.

Weiss, R. S. (ed.) *Loneliness: The experiences of emotional and social isolation*. MIT, Cambridge, MA, 1973.

Williams, L. M. A concept of loneliness in the elderly. *Journal of the American Geriatric Society*. 1978, *24*, 183-187.

Woodward, H., Gingles, R., & Woodward, J. C. Loneliness and the elderly as related to housing. *Gerontologist*, 1974, *14*, 349-351.

Constraints on Leisure Involvement in the Later Years

Francis A. McGuire

ABSTRACT. Leisure is limited by the extent to which constraints constricting leisure choices exist. A study was conducted to examine the constraints which limit leisure behavior in the later years. The results indicated that factors do exist which inhibit leisure choices and the types of constraints to leisure vary across the age groups studied. Leisure service providers must focus more of their efforts on the identification and elimination of such constraints and less on the actual provision of recreation activities if leisure opportunities are to be increased.

Increased longevity and the phenomenon of retirement have resulted in what Michelon (1954) labeled "the new leisure class." The presumed existence of this group is based on the assumption that the free time which accompanies the later years is sufficient to assure a leisure lifestyle. However, this may not be the case. Time may be the essence of leisure, as Brightbill (1960) wrote, but it alone is not sufficient. There must also be freely chosen activities to engage in during that time. Opportunities must exist from which to choose during that time. Conditions which restrict choice will limit leisure in the later years.

In examining the leisure of the elderly, or of any group, it is necessary to expand the focus beyond free time and the activities done during that time. It is essential to investigate perceived freedom and factors limiting that freedom. As Kelly (1982) wrote, "leisure is activity chosen primarily for its own sake." Any force which limits choice limits leisure. The presence of large amounts of unobligated time indicate potential exists for older people to compose a leisure class. However, if the options and alternatives

---

Francis McGuire, PhD, is an assistant professor in the Department of Recreation and Park Administration at Clemson University, Clemson, South Carolina 29631.

An earlier version of this paper was presented at the 1979 National Recreation and Park Association Annual Convention, New Orleans, October, 1979.

17

available during this time are diminished by factors such as biological decline, economic hardship, or social losses, then the existence of the new leisure class may be illusory.

Kalish (1979) cited several reasons why old age may be a time of *increased* freedom of choice. He stated that older people are freed from many responsibilities, such as child rearing and work, which previously impinged on freedom of choice. In addition, older people experience a reduced need to be constrained by what others think of them and, therefore, have the opportunity to step outside the fences that circled their lives. Other reasons for increased freedom of choice, according to Kalish, included: Many older people have worked through fears of their own death and, therefore, have learned how to develop priorities that satisfy them; many older people have large amounts of free time; they are motivated by knowledge that the future is finite and, therefore, are able to focus on things that matter to them. However, other gerontologists do not share Kalish's optimism. They see old age as a time of constriction of choice opportunities. Atchley (1977) stated that freedom of choice in the later years is constricted by physical, financial, and transportation factors. Goldman (1971) suggested that loss of choice is one measure of aging.

Limited research has been done into constraints which may limit leisure in the later years. Trela and Simmons (1971) and Harris (1976) gathered data on factors limiting involvement in senior centers. McAvoy (1976), DeGroot (1976), and Scott and Zoernick (1977) studied factors constraining involvement in a wide range of leisure activities. These studies indicated that the following constrained leisure participation: poor health; lack of transportation; lack of facilities; lack of time; lack of companions; lack of money; fear of crime; physical barriers; lack of skill; feeling too old to learn new activities; and the weather. McAvoy (1976), DeGroot (1976), and Scott and Zoernick (1977) found that the types of constraints experienced by individuals in their later years were different for older respondents than for younger ones. Health and lack of transportation were more salient to the elderly while time and money were more important to younger individuals.

The question of whether the increased free time of old age is accompanied by increased freedom of choice which is necessary to give rise to a new leisure class is one which merits further study. This study expands on previous efforts by examining more potential constraints than prior research. If factors exist which limit choice and, therefore, deprive individuals of leisure opportunities, they must be identified and removed. Therefore, this study was done to answer the following questions:

1. What constraints limit freedom of choice in the later years?
2. Do the types of leisure constraints experienced by older individuals differ from those experienced by younger ones?

PARTICIPANTS AND PROCEDURES

A two-stage sampling design utilized by Lee and Finney (1977) was modified for use with telephone interviews. As a result, 125 individuals residing in a midwestern city were interviewed. They ranged in age from 45 to 93 with a mean age of 63.7. Telephone interviews were used to solicit information about leisure involvement and constraints to involvement. (See McGuire, 1979, and McGuire, 1980, for a detailed report of the sampling procedures and interview schedule.)

Descriptive statistics were used to identify the number and types of constraints experienced by the respondents. Cross-tabulations were used to determine whether the constraints to leisure were different for the younger respondents than for the older respondents.

CONSTRAINTS TO LEISURE INVOLVEMENT

The interviewees identified an average of 9.59 constraints which limited their choice of leisure activities. Lack of time was the most important limiting factor. Over 68% of the respondents reported that time was either somewhat important or very important in preventing participation in desired activities. Eight other constraints were important to at least 40% of the respondents. These included: the weather; lack of money; having more important things to do; being too busy with other activities; lack of energy; being too busy with work; health reasons; and lack of leisure companions. Eight constraints were salient to fewer than 20% of the respondents. These included: feeling that family and friends would not approve of leisure involvement; guilt feelings about leisure participation; not getting a feeling of accomplishment from leisure involvement; and not being good at the activities. Table 1 lists the 30 constraints examined in this study and the number and percentage of respondents identifying each as "not important," "somewhat important," or "very important" in limiting leisure activities.

TABLE 1

PERCENTAGE AND FREQUENCY OF RESPONDENTS NAMING EACH CONSTRAINT
AS "NOT IMPORTANT", "SOMEWHAT IMPORTANT", OR "VERY IMPORTANT"
IN LIMITING LEISURE INVOLVEMENT

Constraint	Not Important	Somewhat Important	Very Important
Not having enough time	31.2%(39)	31.2%(39)	37.6%(47)
The weather	32.0%(40)	34.4%(43)	33.6%(42)
Not having enough money	41.6%(52)	29.6%(37)	28.8%(36)
Having more important things to do	46.4%(58)	28.8%(36)	24.8%(31)
Being too busy with other activities	50.4%(63)	23.2%(29)	26.4%(33)
Lack of energy	52.0%(65)	29.6%(37)	18.4%(23)
Being too busy with work	55.2%(69)	12.0%(15)	32.8%(41)
Health reasons	55.2%(69)	16.0%(20)	28.8%(36)
Not having anyone to do them with	60.0%(75)	22.4%(28)	17.6%(22)
Not having the skills needed	61.6%(77)	22.4%(28)	16.0%(20)
Lack of equipment	63.2%(79)	20.8%(26)	16.0%(20)
Lack of facilities	63.2%(79)	22.4%(28)	14.4%(18)
Friends don't do them	68.0%(85)	24.8%(31)	7.2%(9)
Not knowing how to do them	69.6%(87)	20.8%(26)	9.6%(12)
Feeling too old to learn the activity	69.6%(87)	19.2%(24)	11.2%(14)
Fear of getting hurt	70.4%(88)	13.6%(17)	16.0%(20)
The amount of planning required	73.6%(92)	20.0%(25)	6.4%(8)
Not wanting to interrupt daily schedule	74.4%(93)	16.8%(21)	8.8%(11)

TABLE 1 continued

Constraint	Not Important	Somewhat Important	Very Important
Not having anyone to teach the activities	74.4%(93)	15.2%(19)	10.4%(13)
Too many family responsibilities	76.0%(95)	7.2%(9)	16.8%(21)
Lack of information	76.0%(95)	16.8%(21)	7.2%(9)
Fear of crime	78.4%(98)	8.0%(10)	13.6%(17)
Being no good at the activities	81.6%(102)	14.4%(18)	4.0%(5)
Not getting a feeling of accomplishment	82.4%(103)	12.0%(15)	5.6%(7)
Lack of transportation	83.2%(104)	7.2%(9)	9.6%(12)
Having to make too many decisions	84.0%(105)	12.8%(16)	3.2%(4)
Fear of making a mistake	88.8%(111)	7.2%(9)	4.0%(5)
Feeling guilty about doing them	93.6%(117)	4.8%(6)	1.6%(2)
Fear that others would make fun of participation	93.6%(117)	4.8%(6)	1.6%(2)
Feeling that family and friends would not approve	95.2%(119)	2.4%(3)	2.4%(3)

The respondents were broken into groups on the basis of age (45-59) years of age, 60-74, and 75 or older). The number of interviewees in each age group identifying each constraint as being "not important," "somewhat important," or "very important" was tabulated. Chi-square analysis used to determine whether a significant ($p < .05$) association existed between age and the types of constraints experienced by the study participants. It was found that the factors limiting leisure involvement did vary across the age groups studied. Eleven of the thirty constraints were found to be significantly ($p < .05$) related to age. Seven constraints were more important to the older respondents than to the younger ones. These included: lack of leisure companions; fear of crime; feeling too old to learn new activities; health reasons; lack of transportation; not getting a feeling of accomplishment from leisure participation; and a feeling that family and friends would not approve. Lack of time, being too busy with work, having too many family responsibilities, and having more important things to do were significantly ($p < .05$) more important to the younger respondent than to the older ones in limiting leisure involvement. Although significantly related to age, some of these constraints were important to fewer than 20% of the respondents and should be viewed with caution. These relatively unimportant constraints were lack of transportation, not getting a feeling of accomplishment, and family and friends not approving of leisure participation.

IMPLICATIONS FOR SERVICE DELIVERY

Leisure resides in two worlds: the world of time and the world of perceived freedom. Researchers examining leisure behavior in the later years have been primarily concerned with the first of these. The belief that large amounts of unobligated time can be translated into a leisure lifestyle dominates the traditional mode of thinking. However, free time is only one condition necessary for leisure. Individuals must also perceive opportunities to use that time in desired ways. Any factor which limits that perception reduced the likelihood of entering into a leisure lifestyle.

The respondents in this study identified several constraints which limited their leisure opportunities. It was found that the older respondents were experiencing different types of constraints than their younger counterparts. As Kalish (1979) suggested, constraints primarily related to the roles and obligations of middle age were less salient to the older respondents. As work and family responsibilities decreased, more time became available for leisure. Unfortunately, this increased availability of unobligated time was accompanied by constraints which were not a concern during middle age. The older respondents experienced more constraints related to the social and physical losses associated with the aging process. Since the data in this study were cross sectional in nature, it is impossible to state whether the changing pattern in leisure constraints across the age groups studied reflect a change brought about by the aging process or merely an age difference brought about by something other than the aging process. However, the conclusion that the data reflect an age change is supported by the logical assumption that increasing age is accompanied by role losses which increase the likelihood that constraints such as health, transportation, lack of companions, and fear of crime become more important.

The constraints experienced by the younger respondents, such as being too busy with family or work, are at least partly chosen by the individual. He chooses to invest time in these activities rather than in leisure. However, the constraints which were more important to the older respondents, such as lack of transportation, poor health, lack of leisure companions, fear of crime, and not getting a feeling of accomplishment are factors imposed by forces beyond the control of the individual. These constraints can be removed, or their impact lessened, only by the intervention of outside agents. A function of the individuals involved in the delivery of leisure services, therefore, is to assist in the identification and removal of leisure constraints. They must help potential participants recognize and eliminate factors which narrow freedom of choice and limit leisure opportunities.

The provision of recreational activities is only one step in the delivery of leisure services. If external constraints, such as lack of facilities, lack of equipment, lack of leisure companions, or lack of money, limit leisure involvement, the leisure service provider must assist potential participants by either finding needed resources, providing missing resources, or aiding in the selection of alternate activities. If attitudinal constraints, including not getting a feeling of accomplishment from leisure participation, feeling too old to learn new activities, or feeling that family and friends would not approve of leisure involvement, limit leisure opportunities, it may be necessary to institute a program of leisure counseling to help remove them. If individuals lack the knowledge and skills needed to participate in desired activities, then the leisure service provider must assist in the learning of such skills. With this perspective comes a change in the role of the leisure service provider. No longer is the emphasis on deciding what activities are "appropriate" for individuals participating in a program and then providing only those activities. Rather, the focus shifts to factors limiting leisure choices and the removal of those constraints. In this way the individual is helped to make his own choices. The result of such an altered perspective on the role of the leisure service provider is the maximization of leisure opportunities rather than their constriction.

Constraints which restrict leisure in the later years reduce the likelihood that a large leisure class composed of the elderly can exist. Some individuals live in settings which are conducive to a life of leisure. For example, the leisure emphasis in many retirement communities has fostered a limited leisure class. However, restrictions such as those detailed in this paper prevent many individuals from choosing the leisure alternative in the later years. The promise of a leisure class remains unfulfilled. Until individuals involved in the delivery of leisure services expand their role, it will remain so.

Leisure is one of the few areas in which many older individuals can make their own choices. As other roles are lost, opportunities to exercise control over the environment diminish. This increases the urgency of eliminating factors which reduce perceived freedom of choice in leisure. Doing so assures control over a major sphere of human behavior. The mandate for the individual involved in providing leisure services is clear—create environments where leisure choices are maximized by helping individuals remove constraints which limit opportunities to make their own choices.

REFERENCES

Atchley, R. C. *The social forces in later life*. Belmont: Wadsworth, 1977.

Brightbill, C. K. *The challenge of leisure*. Englewood Cliffs: Prentice-Hall, 1960.

DeGroot, W. L. Analysis of leisure time profiles of selected adult males. Doctoral dissertation, Arizona State University, 1976.

Goldman, S. Social aging, disengagement and loss of choice. *The Gerontologist*, 1971, *11*, 158-162.

Harris, L. *The Myth and Reality of Aging In America*. Washington, D.C.: The National Council on Aging, 1976.

Kalish, R. A. The new ageism and the failure models: A Polemic. *The Gerontologist*, 1979, *19*, 398-402.

Kelly, J. R. *Leisure*. Englewood Cliffs: Prentice-Hall, 1982.

Lee, G. R., & Finney, J. M. Sampling in social gerontology: A method of locating specialized populations. *Journal of Gerontology*, 1977, *32*, 689-693.

McAvoy, L. H. Recreation preferences of elderly persons in Minnesota. Doctoral dissertation, University of Minnesota, 1976.

McGuire, F. A. An exploratory study of leisure constraints in advanced adulthood. Doctoral dissertation, University of Illinois, 1979.

McGuire, F. A. The incongruence between actual and desired leisure involvement in advanced adulthood. *Activities, Adaptation, and Aging*, 1980,*1*(1), 77-89.

Michelon, L. C. The new leisure class. *American Journal of Sociology*, 1954, *59*, 371-378.

Scott, E. O., & Zoernick, D. A. Exploring leisure needs of the aged. *Leisurability*, 1977, *4*, 25-31.

Trella, J. E., & Simmons, R. W. Health and other factors affecting membership and attrition in a senior citizen center. *Journal of Gerontology*, 1971, *26*, 46-51.

Differential Living Arrangements among the Elderly and Their Subjective Well-Being

Charles H. Mindel
Roosevelt Wright, Jr.

ABSTRACT. Attitude literature has consistently shown that the elderly and their children do not desire to share households, preferring "intimacy at a distance." In spite of this, significant numbers of elderly continue to live with relatives. The objective of this study was to examine if elderly living with kin suffer lower morale than elderly living alone or with a spouse. Variables such as race, health, socioeconomic status, and sex, which have been shown to affect morale, were controlled, permitting assessment of the independent effect of living arrangement on morale.

Using multiple classification and analysis of covariance on a random sample of 1332 elderly, race, sex, socioeconomic status and health were found to be significant predictors of morale. After partialing, living arrangement remained a significant predictor of morale. Elderly living with their spouses had the highest level of morale followed by elderly living alone and by elderly living with children. These results indicate that the concerns expressed in negative attitudes toward sharing households with children tend to be borne out once the elderly person shares the household.

During the past forty years a substantial body of research has been amassed concerning life satisfaction, morale and subjective well-being among older people (Tobin and Neugarten, 1961; Edwards and Klemmack, 1973; Medley, 1976; Wolk and Telleen, 1976; Larson, 1978; Hess and Markson, 1980). Much of this research involves relating sociodemographic and social-psycho-

Charles H. Mindel, PhD is Professor, Graduate School of Social Work, The University of Texas at Arlington, Arlington, Texas 76019. Roosevelt Wright, Jr., PhD is Associate Professor, Graduate School of Social Work, The University of Texas at Arlington, Texas 76019.

This article is the revision of a paper presented at the 34th Annual Meeting of the Gerontological Society of America, November, 1981, Toronto, Canada.

logical characteristics of the individual and some aspect(s) of the person's social environment to some measure of morale, satisfaction with life as a whole, or some facet of life satisfaction such as marital satisfaction (Markides and Martin, 1979). However, in spite of the wealth of studies reporting on the correlates and causes of life satisfaction among older Americans, relatively little is known about the relationship between life satisfaction and aspects of the person's living situation such as type of living arrangements, housing, the availability of transportation, etc.

The few studies that have examined these relationships indicate that life satisfaction or subjective well-being is associated with various aspects of people's living situation. Cutler (1972; 1975), for example, has demonstrated a significant relationship between life satisfaction and the availability of transportation among elderly. He found that persons without transportation had a greater frequency of decline in life satisfaction than among those with transportation. These differences were significant with controls for income, health, age, sex, and location of residence.

Several studies have demonstrated a significant relationship between well-being and housing (Carp, 1968; Schooler, 1970; Smith and Lipman, 1972; Martin, 1973; Lawton and Cohen, 1974). They suggest that differences in housing affect well-being, that is, the physical aspects of a dwelling directly affect a person's subjective assessment of life satisfaction. Two studies, however, did not find an association between well-being and frequency of residential moves (Maddox and Eisdorfer, 1962; Palmore and Luikart, 1972). Thus, although these studies have found a positive relationship between aspects of a person's living situation and life satisfaction, the findings have not been uniformly positive nor have they always found the relationship to be a strong one. As a result, few definite statements may be made about these relationships (Lohmann, 1980).

Living Arrangements

It is clear by now that most elderly in the United States do not live in institutions; over 95 percent are non-institutionalized. The 95 percent of non-institutionalized elderly tend to fall into three major categories: (a) those who live alone, (b) those who live with a spouse, and (c) those who live with kin. While the number of institutionalized elderly has not changed substantially over the last generation or so there have been major changes in the types of living arrangements of the remaining large majority. For example, since

1940 in the United States the proportion of elderly men who live with their kin has declined from approximately 15 percent to 4 percent in 1975. For women the decline in the number of elderly women living with kin has declined from 30 percent to 13 percent over the same 35 years. However, the proportion of "single" elderly (i.e., unmarried, no longer married) living with relatives had reached a relatively stable 30-35 percent throughout the 1970s (Mindel, 1979).

With respect to those elderly who live with their spouses, definite changes are found. In 1965, 68 percent of elderly males lived with their spouses compared to 74 percent in 1975. For elderly females the figures are quite different; 34 percent were living with a spouse in 1965 compared to 23 percent in 1975 (Mindel, 1979; Siegel, 1976).

The changes among those living alone are more substantial for women than men, with 29 percent of elderly women living alone in 1965 compared to 36 percent in 1975. For men the shift was from 13 percent in 1965 to 14 percent in 1975 (Mindel, 1979; Siegel, 1976).

It has been suggested in various studies that elderly who are living with their children tend to be older (Hess and Markson, 1980; Riley and Foner, 1968), female (Kivett and Learner, 1980; Seelbach, 1977; Hendricks and Hendricks, 1977), less affluent (Donahue et al., 1969; Beresford and Rivlin, 1969), come from ethnic and minority groups (Mindel, 1975; Hess and Markson, 1980; Kosa et al., 1970; Cantor, 1976; Troll, 1971; Lee, 1980), are in poorer health (National Health Survey, 1960; Shanas, 1979; Troll, 1971), have closer ties to kin (Mindel, 1975; Shanas, 1979; Kosa et al., 1960), and are more isolated and lonely than elderly in other living arrangements (Smith et al., 1975; Donahue et al., 1969; Kivett and Learner, 1980). Moreover, it has been argued that those elderly who are married tend to be younger, white, wealthier, have better perceptions of themselves, are in better health, and participate more in organizations and with friends (Hess and Markson, 1980; Kobrin and Hendershot, 1977; Lee, 1978; Morgan, 1976).

Elderly living alone tend to fall somewhere between the elderly living with children and elderly living with their spouse on many of these characteristics. Since many are widows they tend to be older, have less money, and be in poorer health than the married. They are reasonably close to their relatives and are socially active (Hess and Markson, 1980; Morgan, 1976; Shanas, 1979; Lopata, 1973; Lee, 1978; Kobrin and Hendershot, 1977; Atcheley, 1975).

The different types of living arrangements as they might affect morale, conceptually might be thought of as indicators of two social-psychological dimensions, "autonomy" and "involvement/isolation" (Mindel, 1981). It has been found that elderly who live with their spouses were more autonomous and less dependent and less isolated than elderly who live with a child, who were more likely to be dependent and socially isolated. Elderly who live alone were found to fall near the elderly with spouse on involvement and nearer the elderly living with children on autonomy (Mindel, 1981).

It is expected that high morale should be related to high autonomy and high involvement and that low morale should be related to high dependency and high isolation. Thus we hypothesize that the elderly living with children will have the lowest morale, the elderly living with their spouses the highest, and the elderly living alone will be found between the two of them.

In an attempt to examine the effects of living arrangements rather than other potentially confounding variables such as age, sex, race, income and health, an analysis of covariance model will be presented in which the effects of confounding variables will be removed, permitting an assessment of the unique effects of living arrangements.

METHODS

Sample

This study represents a secondary analysis of a study entitled "The Study of Well Being of Older People in Cleveland, Ohio: 1975-1976." The data were furnished by the Inter-University Consortium for Political and Social Research. The original study in Cleveland was a random probability sample of 1834 non-institutionalized elderly people aged 65 or over. In this analysis 1332 of the 1834 cases will be analyzed. The 502 missing cases were lost due to missing information on one or more of the variables.

Some of the descriptive characteristics of this sample are as follows: 69 percent of the sample was white and 31 percent was black; 64 percent were female and 36 percent were male. The median age of the respondents in this analysis was 72.5 years and the median income was $3,500. Of the 1332 individuals in the three types of living arrangement, 592 or 44 percent lived alone, 442 or 33.2 percent lived with a spouse, and 298 or 22.4 percent of the sample lived with a child.

Measurement

The primary independent variable, living arrangement, was measured by coding the response to several questions concerning who lived with the respondent. If the respondent answered no one, they were categorized as living alone, if they answered with their husband or wife, they were categorized as living with a spouse and if they stated that a child lived with them they were put into that category. Individuals who lived with a spouse and a child were put into the living with spouse category rather than the living with child category. The covariates, age, race, sex, and income, were coded in the standard way. Health was measured on a 4-point self-rated scale ranging from excellent to poor. Morale, the dependent variable, was measured using the Duke University Mental Health Multi-dimensional Functional Assessment Questionnaire's scale (Pfeiffer, 1975). The mental health scale consists of 15 questions regarding various mental health symptoms. This sample, however, presented a somewhat restricted range of responses. The scale score ranges from 0 to 15 symptoms. The mean score on this sample was 3.15, indicating a relatively high level of well-being as measured by the scale.

Statistical Analysis

The method of analysis used in this study was analysis of covariance and multiple classification analysis. The purpose of these techniques is to partial out the effects of the covariates (age, race, sex, income, and health) which have been shown in the past to be significant predictors of morale. An examination of the unique effects and contributions of living arrangements on the measure of morale can then be made. In addition, the multiple classification analysis is a method by which a set of means, in this case the mean morale scores, can be estimated which represent the differences between the three living arrangement types after they have been adjusted for the effects of the covariates.

RESULTS

The analysis of covariance presented in Table 1 indicates that except for age all covariates were significant at the .01 level or less. After partialing out the effects of these covariates it was found that living arrangements was also significant at the .01 level. The six variables accounted for 31.5 percent of the non-error variance in morale. By far the best predictor was health, which explained 23.5 percent of the variance.

In Table 2 estimates of the mean morale scores for the three groups both before and after adjustments have been made for the covariates are presented. The results indicate that the elderly who live with their spouses had the highest morale, followed by those who lived alone and lastly by the elderly who lived with their children. This holds true both before and after adjustments were made for the covariates. After adjustments were made for the covariates the differences between the three groups declined somewhat, with the elderly living with their spouses being at one extreme and the elderly living alone or with children being grouped somewhat together at the other. However, since the morale scores range from 0 through 15, it cannot be said that morale was generally very low for any of the three groups.

TABLE 1

Analysis of Covariance of Selected

Characteristics Related to Morale*

Source of Variation	Sum of Squares	df	Mean Square	F	P
Covariates					
Age	9.78	1	9.78	1.57	.21
Race	38.16	1	38.16	6.11	.01
Sex	67.15	1	67.15	10.75	.001
Income	92.77	1	92.77	14.85	.0001
Health	2839.78	1	2839.78	454.45	.0001
Main Effect					
Living Arrangements	56.84	2	28.42	4.55	.01
Residual	8273.40	1324	6.25		
Total	12071.76	1331			

*R^2 = .315

TABLE 2

Multiple Classification Analysis of Covariates

& Independent Variable with Morale

Living Arrangement	N	Unadjusted Means	Means Adjusted for Covariates & Independent Variable
Lives alone	592	3.34	3.19
Lives with spouse	442	2.40	2.86
Lives with child(ren)	298	3.89	3.49

DISCUSSION

In this study of 1332 elderly it was hypothesized that the environmental situation (living arrangements) in which an elderly person found him or herself would affect the morale or subjective well-being of that person. It had been expected that those elderly living with their spouses would have the highest morale and that those elderly living with their children would have the lowest morale. In order to remove the confounding effects of health, age, income, race, and sex, which have often been confounding factors in examining the effects of living arrangement, an analysis of covariance was run which partialed out these effects. It was found that after removing the effects of the covariates, living arrangement still contributed a statistically significant amount of the variance in morale.

The initial hypotheses were predicted upon the premise that elderly living with children were more likely to be dependent and isolated and thus would have lower morale; that elderly living with a spouse were likely to be autonomous and involved and thus have higher morale; and that elderly living alone would fall somewhere in between. These patterns were found both before and after partialing out the effects of the control variables. The relatively small percentage of the variance that living arrangement explains can perhaps be explained in terms of the model proposed here. That is, dependency may be linked not so much with living arrangement but with such matters as health and income (the two most important variables in this analysis). Limitations of health and income restrict autonomy and involvement and thus reduce morale. Living arrangement type independent of income and health also relates to autonomy and involvement but is not nearly as strong a factor. That it is still significant after partialing reflects the importance of the environmental component in understanding morale. Nevertheless, the data here clearly demonstrate that the best predictor of morale is the individual characteristic of self-perceived health status.

Implications

Although living arrangements were found to be a statistically significant predictor of morale among the non-institutionalized elderly, it does not appear to be a powerful one, accounting for approximately one percent of the non-error variance. This finding, however, tends to confirm much of the literature and research concerning elderly who live with children as well as elderly in other living arrangements (Troll, 1971). A possible explanation for this observation is that large numbers of elderly remain in their own home with children and other kin joining their households. This arrangement, in general, is more conducive to producing higher levels of morale among the elderly than the reverse (Mindel, 1979; Kivett and Learner, 1982).

The finding that health status is the most important predictor of subjective well-being is consistent with the existing literature (Markides and Martin, 1979; Lohmann, 1980). Good health is known to be associated with higher levels of satisfaction in later life.

The importance of health to the subjective well-being of the elderly has important implications for the formulation of future social policies and programs. The current health status of the elderly is subject to relatively little, if any, socially acceptable policy manipulation. Thus for the present generation of older Americans there is probably very little that can be done to change their health status through social policies. We can only hope that the provision of health care and social services to them will minimize the debilitating effect of health conditions and thus prevent further declines in subjective well-being or morale (Lohmann, 1980). Our best chances of influencing health through social policies is to focus our attention on the current generations of younger people (the future aged) by developing comprehensive and early screening, identification, and diagnostic health programs that emphasize preventive health care and education. These efforts may produce further generations of older people whose health contributes in positive ways to their morale or subjective well-being.

In conclusion, the findings from the present study indicate that the kinds of living arrangements in which non-institutionalized elderly people are involved are not major risks to their subjective well-being. The morale of the elderly is strongly associated with such factors as health status, financial and economic inadequacy, restricted autonomy, social isolation, etc., which may result in an older person needing a certain type of living arrangement for survival, maintenance, and care. As a result, efforts must be made to provide adequate economic and social services to those who have assumed responsibility for the maintenance and care of dependent older people—their children, relatives, and friends.

REFERENCES

Atchley, R. Dimensions of widowhood in later life. *The Gerontologist,* 1975, *15,* 176-178.

Beresford, J. C. and Rivlin, A. The multigenerational family, in W. Donohue, J. L. Kornbluh, and L. Power (eds.), *Living in the multigenerational family.* Institute of Gerontology, University of Michigan - Wayne State University, 1969, 1-36.

Cantor, M. The Configuration and intensity of the informal support system in a New York City elderly population. Paper presented at the 29th Annual meeting of the Gerontological Society, New York, 1976.

Carp, F. Effects of improved housing on the lives of older people. In B. N. Neugarten (ed.), *Middle age and aging.* University of Chicago Press, Chicago, 1968.

Cutler, S. The availability of personal transportation, residential location, and life satisfaction among the aged. *Journal of Gerontology,* 1972, *27,* 383-389.

Cutler, S. Transportation and changes in life satisfaction. *Gerontologist,* 1975, *15,* 155-159.

Donahue, W., Kornbluh, J. L., and Power, L. (eds.), *Living in the multigenerational family.* Institute of Gerontology, University of Michigan - Wayne State University, 1969.

Edwards, J., and Klemmack, D. Correlates of life satisfaction; A reexamination. *Journal of Gerontology,* 1973, *28,* 497-502.

Hendricks, J., and Hendricks, C. D., *Aging in mass society: Myths and realities.* Cambridge, MA: Winthrop, 1977.

Hess, B. B., and Markson, E. W. *Aging and old age,* New York; Macmillan, 1980.

Kivett, V. R., and Learner, R. M. Situational influences on the morale of older rural adults in child-shared housing: A comparative analysis. *Gerontologist,* 1982, *22,* 100-106.

Kobrin, F. E., and Hendershot, G. E. Do family ties reduce mortality? Evidence from the United States 1966-1968, *Journal of Marriage and the Family,* 1977, *39,* 737-746.

Kosa, J., Rachiele, L. D., and Schommer, C. O. Sharing the home with relatives. *Marriage and Family Living,* 1970, *22,* 129-131.

Lawton, M., and Cohen, J. The generality of housing impact on the well-being of older people. *Journal of Gerontology,* 1974, *29,* 194-204.

Lee, G. L. Kinship in the seventies. *Journal of Marriage and the Family,* 1980, *42,* 923-934.

Lee, G. R. Marriage and morale in later life. *Journal of Marriage and Development,* 1976, *7,* 107-115.

Lopata, H. *Widowhood in an American city.* Cambridge, MA: Schenckman, 1973.

Lohmann, N. Life satisfaction research in aging: Implications for policy development, in Datan, N., and Lohmann, N. (eds.), *Transitions of aging,* NY: Academic Press, 1980.

Maddox, G., and Eisdorfer, C. Some correlates of activity and morale among the elderly. *Social Forces,* 1962, *41,* 254-260.

Markides, K. S., and Martin, H. W. A causal model of life satisfaction among the elderly. *Journal of Gerontology*, 1979, *34*, 86-93.

Martin, W. Activity and disengagement: Life satisfaction of in-movers into a retirement community. *Gerontologist*, 1973, *13*, 224-227.

Medley, M. Satisfaction with life among persons sixty-five years or older: A causal model. *Journal of Gerontology*, 1976, *31*, 448-455.

Mindel, C. H. Multigenerational family living: A viable alternative for the aged in industrial society. Paper read at 10th International Congress of Gerontology, Jerusalem, Israel, 1975.

Mindel, C. H. Multigenerational family households: Recent trends and implications for the future. *The Gerontologist*, 1979, *19*, 456-463.

Mindel, C. H. Characteristics of the elderly in three types of living arrangements. Paper presented at the XII International Congress of Gerontology, Hamburg, W. Germany, 1981.

Morgan, L. A reexamination of widowhood and morale. *Journal of Gerontology*, 1976, *31*, 687-695.

National Health Survey, Older persons, selected health characteristics, United States, July 1957-July 1959, Series C4—Publication No. 584. Washington, D.C.: Government Printing Office, 1960.

Palmore, E., and Luikart, C. Health and social factors related to life satisfaction. *Journal of Gerontology*, 1961, *16*, 134-143.

Pfeiffer, E. *Functional assessment: The OARS Multidimensional function assessment questionnaire*. Duke University Center, Durham, NC, 1975.

Riley, M. W., and Foner, A. Aging and society, vol. 1: An inventory of cycle. *Journal of Marriage and the Family*, 1970, *32*, 20-28.

Schooler, K. Effect of environment on morale. *Gerontologist*, 1970, *10*, 194-197.

Seelbach, W. Gender differences in expectations of filial responsibility. *The Gerontologist*, 1977, *17*, 421-425.

Shanas, E. The family as a social support system in old age. *The Gerontologist*, 1979, *19*, 169-174.

Siegel, J. S. Demographic aspects of aging and the older population in the United States. *Current Population Efforts*, Special Studies, series P-23, no. 59, 1976.

Smith, K., and Lipman, A. Constraint and life satisfaction. *Journal of Gerontology*, 1972, *27*, 77-82.

Smith, W. M., Britton, J. H., and Britton, J. O. *Relationships within three generation families*. University Park, PA: The Pennsylvania State University Press.

Tobin, S., and Neugarten, B. Life satisfaction and social interaction in the aging. *Journal of Gerontology*, 1961, 344-346.

Troll, L. E. The family of later life: A decade review. *Journal of Marriage and the Family*, 1971, *33*, 263-290.

Wolk, S., and Telleen, S. Psychological and social correlates of life satisfaction as a function of residential constraint. *Journal of Gerontology*, 1976, *31*, 89-98.

Determinants of Life Satisfaction among Black Elderly

V. V. Prakasa Rao
V. Nandini Rao

ABSTRACT. The paper examines the relative influence of social, economic, health and familial variables in explaining the sex differences in the life satisfaction of the black elderly. The dependent variable was measured using the life satisfaction Index A scale on a sample of 240 retired individuals living in a Southern metropolitan area. Multiple regression analysis revealed that nearly 52 percent of variance in life satisfaction for males was explained by all (24) independent variables while only 19 percent of variance in the dependent variable for females was explained by the same independent variables. The stepwise regression analysis yielded a six-variable optimal model for life satisfaction for males while a two-variable model was found for females. It is suggested that additional research be conducted to determine if this difference exists in other populations and samples of the black elderly.

The Life Satisfaction Index developed by Neugarten, Havighurst and Tobin (1961) is probably the most extensively used and well established measure of life satisfaction. Since the development of the LSIA scale life satisfaction has become a central research topic for study in the aging process. Most of the existing research on life satisfaction can be classified into two types: (1) the studies mainly dealing with identification of significant variables associated with life satisfaction and/or determination of predictor variables of life

V.V. Prakasa Rao, PhD is Professor, Department of Sociology and Faculty Fellow, Research Institute for Socio-Technical Problems, Jackson State University, Jackson, MS 39217. V. Nandini Rao, PhD is Professor, Department of Sociology, Jackson State University, Jackson, MS 39217.

This is a revised version of a paper presented at the meeting of the XII International Congress of Gerontology, Hamburg, West Germany, August, 1981. Analysis of the paper was made possible in part by the Charles Stewart Mott Foundation. The views contained in this publication do not necessarily reflect those of the Mott Foundation, its trustees, or officers. Thanks are extended to James Brooks for comments and suggestions on the earlier version of the paper.

35

satisfaction among predominantly white elderly; and (2) the studies primarily concerned with comparing different groups on the basis of race, ethnicity, sex, age, and residence. It should be noted, however, that substantial differences are found in the levels of life satisfaction between blacks and whites.

Comparative studies based on race derive their justification from the argument that the life experiences and the situational factors affecting the minority aged are different from those of white elderly. Added impetus is also given by the argument that the plight of the black elderly has been described as one of "double jeopardy" (Jackson, 1971; National Urban League, 1964). The black aged are said to bear a double burden which has a negative effect of being *old* and *black*. Research comparing differences in life satisfaction is very limited. The available research indicated that the findings with respect to race are not only inconclusive but they are often contradictory. Alston et al. (1972) found that blacks tend to express lower levels of life satisfaction than whites. In contrast, Messer (1968) observed considerably higher levels of life satisfaction among blacks. In one of the most recent studies, Donnenwerth et al. (1978) found that whites had a significantly higher mean life satisfaction score than blacks. When controlled for residence, life satisfaction was higher among rural blacks and urban whites compared to their counterparts. Sauer (1977) found a significant relationship between race and morale with blacks scoring higher on morale than whites. However, race proved to be an inefficient predictor of morale when the regression analysis was performed. Clemente and Sauer (1974) and Spreitzer and Snyder (1974) found no differences in life satisfaction between white and black elderly. The preceding review of literature indicates inconclusive empirical evidence with regard to life satisfaction on the basis of race.

As mentioned earlier, since black elderly experience unique life events it is assumed that their aging process and service needs are different from the dominant group. Moore (1971) listed five characteristics relevant for the aging process of all minorities. (1) Each minority has a *special history* which is not only different from the white population but also entails subordination. In the case of blacks. slavery and its aftermath placed them into a different collective experience. (2) The special history has been accompanied by *discrimination* and the development of negative stereotypes about blacks. (3) Most of the minority groups developed *variant subcultures* which include values and norms relative to behaviors in different age groups. (4) Once the subcultures enabled them to learn bare survival techniques in relation to fulfilling basic needs, to engage in meaningful social participation, *internal prestige and power,* and to provide opportunity for a sense of belonging to some collectivity. (5) Finally, although things have been *changing rapidly,* exploitation, discrimination and prejudice still continue (Moore, 1971: 88-89). Jackson (1972) also points out how black aged are different from white aged. She observed (1972:32) that "in so far as black old people are concerned, I think that we should not begin to treat them as if they were the same as white old people. They are not. Racism has adversely affected their preparation for old age."

In spite of a great deal of research in the area of life satisfaction, with one exception (Jackson et al., 1977), no empirical research has been conducted on the black aged population *per se* over the last three decades. The need for empirical data to determine the factors associated with life satisfaction has been emphasized by researchers, social workers, and policy makers. After an extensive review of the literature on minority aging, Jackson (1980:219) still contends that "the current status of research about minority aging is still highly fragmented and inconclusive. More rigorous and sophisticated research is needed, including appropriate mixtures of cross-sectional and longitudinal studies of representative samples of various age cohorts over time."

Failure to study the black aged population as a separate group as well as the differences and similarities between different subgroups based on socioeconomic and demographic characteristics may lead us to ignore the heterogeneous nature of the group. Solomon (1971: 1-2) recognized the importance of this argument when she points out that "it is not consistent with reality to talk about the black aged as if they were a homogeneous group, all having the same kind of life experience and having had the same kind of things happen to them." Jackson (1980: 5-6) also argues forcefully that "the examination of these groups also may make us more aware of the heterogeneity of aging. In a nutshell, the argument here is that older persons do not experience problems solely on the basis of aging."

The only study conducted to examine the determinants of self-reported life satisfaction among blacks was by Jackson et al. (1977). Based on multiple regression analysis, the study found that level of education, self-assessed health, attitudes toward employment of the elderly, attitudes toward intrinsic religiosity, self-esteem and need affiliation to be the strongest variables in explaining variance in life satisfaction among aged blacks. The sixteen variables entered in the multiple regression equation accounted for 41 percent of the variance.

The major purpose of the present research is to examine the relationship between a number of socioeconomic, demographic, familial, and intergenerational mutual help variables and self-reported life satisfaction and to determine the most salient variables in explaining the variance in life satisfaction. Additionally, the factors associated with the predictors of life satisfaction will be determined for the male and female subgroups. It is assumed that even if there are no significant differences between sexes in life satisfaction, it is quite possible that the predictors of life satisfaction for males may be different from females.

METHODS

A sample of 240 elderly blacks residing in noninstitutionalized settings was selected from Jackson, Mississippi which has a population of approximately 300,000. The respondents were selected from different areas of the city where heavy concentrations of black Americans reside. An effort was made to include subjects with different socioeconomic status by collecting information from different neighborhoods. The data were collected in Spring, 1978. The sample contained 41 percent males and 59 percent females. There were 28 percent in the age category under 65; 30 percent, 66-70; 17 percent, 71-75; 13 percent, 76-80; and 12 percent 81 and over.

The dependent variable life satisfaction was measured by the Life Satisfaction Index-A (LISA) developed by Neugarten, Havighurst and Tobin (1961). The 20-item index was tested for validity and item reliability on black elderly and found to be a highly appropriate measure (Rao and Rao, 1982). Hence all the items were retained in the study to measure the life satisfaction of the black elderly.

A total of 24 predictor variables were included in the study to examine their influence on the criterion variable. Age of the respondent was operationalized in terms of the actual age reported at the time of interview. Marital status was coded zero for married and one for divorced, widowed or separated. Education was measured in terms of the actual number of school years completed by the respondent. Income was operationalized on the basis of responses to the question, "What is your and your spouse's monthly income including welfare payment, retirement income, etc. We don't need the exact amount, just give the approximate amount.'' Responses were coded, by $100 intervals, from 1 for $100 and/or less, through 4 for $301 to $400, 7 for $401 to $700 and 11 for $1001 and over. Occupation before retirement was measured by assigning Duncan's Socioeconomic Index scores which range from 00 to 99 to the occupation the respondent indicated. Self-rated health was measured by the question, ''How would you describe your health?'' followed by five responses: ''very poor,'' ''poor,'' ''sometimes good, sometimes not,'' ''good,'' and ''very good.'' Responses were scored from 1 to 5 respectively.

The actual number reported by the respondents was coded to determine the number of sons, the number of daughters, the number of siblings and the number of grandchildren. Responses for living arrangements were coded 1 for ''live with spouse,'' 2 for ''live with daughters, sons, grandchildren, and others,'' and 3 for ''live alone,'' Distance of the nearest child was determined by the question, ''How far do you live from your nearest child?'' The respondents were given six alternatives to respond: ''same house,'' ''10 minutes journey or less,'' ''11-30 minutes,'' ''31 minutes to 1 hour,'' ''over 1 hour but less than 1 day,'' and ''1 day or more.'' The higher the score, the greater the distance to the nearest child. Sex of the nearest child was determined by the response given to this question: ''Is your nearest child a male or female?'' Sex was coded one for males and two for females.

To determine the social interaction measures, the black elderly were asked to respond to nine items. Each item was followed by two responses—yes or no. The following items were used in the study as measures of social interaction.

1. See your children weekly or more often
2. Talk to children by phone weekly or more often
3. See siblings weekly or more often
4. Talk with siblings by phone weekly or more often
5. See grandchildren weekly or more often
6. Talk with grandchildren by phone weekly or more often
7. See close friends weekly or more often
8. Talk with close friends by phone weekly or more often
9. See and visit people as often an you would like

A positive response was scored 2 while a negative response was coded 1.

Intergenerational Exchange of Help Scale developed by Bild and Havighurst (1976) was used in the study to determine the help the elderly received from the children or grandchildren. Intergenerational exchange of help the elderly received was indexed by a nine-item scale. The respondents were asked in the following manner: "Have any of your children or grandchildren provided help in the following areas?"

1. Helped out when either of you were sick
2. Given advice on business or money matters
3. Ever offered you financial assistance
4. Helped you shop
5. Given you a gift
6. Helped fix things around the house
7. Helped you with housekeeping
8. Driven you places you need to go
9. Given advice on life's problems

Each item was scored on a two point response set. An affirmative response was coded 2 while the negative response was accorded a value of 1. The responses for the nine items were summed to create the scale. The higher the score, the greater help the respondents received from their children or grandchildren. To determine the help the elderly provided to their children or grandchildren, eight items were modified to read whether the elderly helped them in the areas mentioned in the scale. Item "Driven you places you need to go" was replaced by "Helped care for their children." A scoring pattern similar to the one used above was also used to measure the help the elderly provided their children and grandchildren.

RESULTS

Zero-order correlations reveal that occupation, income, the number of daughters, the number of grandchildren, the number of siblings, sex of the nearest child, face to face interaction with siblings, talk with siblings over the phone and talk to grandchildren by phone are positively related to the life satisfaction of the total sample while living arrangements is negatively related to the dependent variable. For the male subsample, education, occupation, income, the number of daughters, the number of grandchildren, talking to children and talking to siblings were positively related while age and the number of sons were negatively related to life satisfaction. For the female subsample, income, the number of grandchildren, the number of siblings, sex of the nearest child, seeing siblings, and seeing people were significantly associated with life satisfaction. Based on the zero-order correlations, it is observed that only two independent variables—income and the number of grandchildren—are significantly related to life satisfaction for both sexes while the remaining significant variables are different for males compared to females.

In order to obtain a more precise picture of the relative contribution of each independent variable while the other variables are statistically controlled, a stepwise multiple regression analysis was computed with life satisfaction as a criterion variable for the total sample, and for the subsamples of males and females. This method tends to yield the most significant variables that explain the greatest amount of variance in the dependent variable. The 24 demographic, socioeconomic, familial and social interaction variables formed the item pool from which the "best" models are constructed for the total sample, and the subsamples of males and females.

Table 1 reports the effects of the strongest independent variables on life satisfaction for the total samples, and the male and female subsamples. The optimal model for the total sample is the five-variable model. It indicates that the black elderly who have higher levels of income, report large numbers of grandchildren, talk to grandchildren once a week or more often, see close friends less often, and do not see their children often tend to express greater levels of satisfaction with their lives. The five-variable model explained 18.1 percent of the variance in the criterion variable. From both the standardized regression coefficients (*beta* weights) and the increments in R^2, it is clear that income and the number of grandchildren are the most powerful explanatory variables compared to the remaining three salient variables in the model. In fact, income and the number of grandchildren account for 58 percent and 29 percent of the total explained variance respectively while the other three variables together account for only 13 percent of the total explained variance in life satisfaction. It is also surprising to note that although living arrangement, occupation, number of daughters, number of siblings, sex of the nearest child, talking to siblings, and seeing siblings are correlated with life satisfaction, they do not emerge as significant predictors when the effects of independent variables are removed in

TABLE 1. STEPWISE MULTIPLE REGRESSION OF STRONGEST VARIABLES RELATED TO LIFE SATISFACTION BY SEX*

Variables	Multiple Correlation	Cumulative Variance $(R)^2$	Change in R^2	Beta (Standardized)	Percentage of Explained Variance
		Sample (N = 240)			
Income	.324	.105	.105	.304	58.0
Number of grandchildren	.397	.157	.052	.211	28.7
Talk to grandchildren	.410	.168	.011	.155	6.1
See close friends	.418	.175	.007	-.102	3.9
See children	.425	.181	.006	-.100	3.3
All Independent variables					
Together	.469	.220			
		Males (N = 96)			
Number of grandchildren	.525	.276	.276	.419	59.3
Income	.616	.379	.104	.270	22.3
Age	.638	.407	.028	-.149	6.0
Talk to children	.653	.427	.020	.186	4.2
Number of sons	.669	.448	.021	-.174	4.6
Health	.682	.465	.017	.146	3.6
All Independent Variables					
Together	.719	.516			
		Females (N = 144)			

TABLE 1. (continued)

Variables	Multiple Correlation	Cumulative Variance $(R)^2$	Change in R^2	Beta (Standardized)	Percentage of Explained Variance
See Siblings	.156	.024	.024	.174	47.5
See and Visit People	.227	.051	.027	-.166	52.5
All Independent Variables					
Together	.437	.191			

* Significant at .05 level or beyond.

the multiple regression equations. Equally striking is the fact that although seeing close friends once a week or more often is not significantly related to the dependent variable, the contribution of this variable seems to be strong based on *beta* weights when the effects of other variables are eliminated.

The results of the stepwise multiple regression analysis indicate that a six-variable model is the model of choice for the male subsample. Black elderly males who report large numbers of grandchildren, have higher levels of income, are relatively young, talk to children once a week or more often, have fewer sons and enjoy good health express higher levels of life satisfaction compared to black elderly males who have the opposite qualities. These six variables explain 46.5 percent of the variance in life satisfaction. The effect of number of children on the criterion variable is strong and positive. The level of income also has a fairly substantial effect on life satisfaction. The number of children and income account for 59.3 percent and 22.3 percent of the total explained variance respectively. The other four variables in the regression equation (age, talk to children, number of sons, and health) collectively account for 18.2 percent of the variance. It should be pointed out, however, that although education, occupation, number of daughters and talking to siblings are correlated with life satisfaction, they bear no relationship when influences of other variables are held constant. Surprisingly, health (although the correlation is not significant) appears to be a major contributor in explaining the variance in the dependent variable (*beta* weight = .146).

Finally, the optimal model for the female subsample is a two-variable model. Females, who see siblings once a week or more often and visit people less often, tend to be more satisfied with their lives. It is surprising to note that there are no common variables in the male and female optimal models that explain variance in life satisfaction. The regression model contains two variables for females while it constitutes six variables for males. The optimal model for females explains only 5.1 percent of the variance in the criterion variable. Seeing siblings once a week or more often accounts for 47.5 percent while visiting people as less often as they desire accounts for 52.5 percent of the total variance. Although the correlates of income, the number of grandchildren, see children, and number of siblings with life satisfaction are positive and strong, their independent contributions are negligible when the effects of other variables are eliminated.

SUMMARY AND CONCLUSION

The study was primarily concerned with identifying a number of independent variables associated with life satisfaction as well as determining the most salient variables of satisfaction with life of the black elderly population and also the male and female subsamples. The findings are offered with a note of caution as the sample was mainly regional in nature. The study has presented results from zero-order correlations and step-wise multiple regression analysis. The latter method was used to determine the true contribution of each of the independent variables in explaining variance in life satisfaction.

The optimal models on life satisfaction for the total sample and the male and female subsamples indicate that the most significant variables were different as well as the magnitude of cumulative variance explained by these variables for each of the three groups. When the 24 independent variables were employed to explain variance in life satisfaction for the total sample, the study indicated that 22 percent of the variance was explained. This finding is comparable with 24 percent, 23 percent, 25 percent and 24 percent variance explained by Edwards and Klemmack (1973), Palmore and Luikart (1972), Sauer (1977), and Spreitzer and Synder (1974), respectively, in earlier studies.

The results of this study were somewhat surprising as they varied from the previous research findings in explaining differences in life satisfaction. It should also be mentioned that the comparision of the findings of this study with previous research may be problematic since the number and type of independent variables used in this and other studies are different, also the measures of life satisfaction are not similar. With regard to the total sample, income, number of grandchildren, talking to grandchildren, seeing close friends, and seeing children were the most significant determinants of life satisfaction. The finding that income is the most important variable in explaining life satisfaction corresponds with numerous studies which have established a positive relationship between these two variables (Edwards and Klemmack, 1973; Larson, 1975; Markides and Martin, 1979; Medley, 1976; Palmore and Luikart, 1972). The results also lend support to the previous research that social interaction with friends and kin as well as other familial variables are important in the respondent's life satisfaction. The fact that number of grandchildren and talking to them have turned out to be salient variables could be explained by an argument that black people maintain extended family relations and social contacts with their grandchildren. Kinship research also confirms our findings that black people tend to maintain strong kin ties as indicated by co-residence, visiting, and exchange of mutual help among kin, for the sake of survival in a hostile environment (Allen, 1979; Hayes and Mindel, 1973; McAdoo, 1978; Stack, 1975). However, an unexpected finding was that the more often the black elderly saw their children, the less satisfied they were with their lives. This is surprising given the findings of earlier researchers regarding importance of kinship relations among blacks. It suggests that the mere frequency of interaction with children does not guarantee satisfaction with life for older people. A person can be surrounded by other people but at the same time may be lonely and feel detached. It may be that the quality of interaction is more important than frequency of interaction with children in explaining life satisfaction. It is not how often one interacts with family members but what kind of interaction one establishes that perhaps determines whether the elderly are satisfied or not.

The findings of this study are somewhat puzzling and unexpected with regard to the total explained variance in life satisfaction across gender groups and also the number of determinants of the dependent variable. Six variables emerged as the predictors of life satisfaction for black elderly males, while only two variables emerged as the predictors of life satisfaction for black elderly females. Black males who are relatively less advanced in age, report large number of grandchildren, have high income, talk to children by phone once a week or more often, have a fewer number of sons and have good health tend to express higher levels of life satisfaction. In contrast, females tend to be more satisfied if they see their siblings weekly or more often and do not see and visit people as often as they like. It is apparent that the explanatory variables of the criterion variable are different for the black male and female subsamples.

The data for black males suggests that some determinants—such as income, age, and health—of life satisfaction are consistent with the findings of previous research. The negative relationship between the number of sons and life satisfaction is somewhat unexpected. One of the explanations for this surprising finding may be given by the argument that the sons are expected to fulfill instrumental functions of their fathers such as helping financially as they become older. It is possible for the parents to expect more from their sons which might result in lower satisfaction as their high expectations are not fulfilled.

The amount of difference in explained variance in life satisfaction between the male and female subsamples is an unexpected finding. Nearly 52 percent of the variance in life satisfaction is explained by all 24 variables together for elderly males while only 19 percent of variance in life satisfaction is explained by the same dependent variables for elderly females. Further research might explain the black females' life satisfaction. Only two variables, seeing siblings once a week or more often and visiting friends, emerged as significant predictors of life satisfaction for black elderly females. The finding that face to face interaction with siblings is important for females can be explained by their marital status and living arrangement. Nearly two-thirds of females compared to only one-half of males are either unmarried, divorced, widowed or remained single at the time of the survey. A similar percentage of black females either live alone or with others. It appears that once they are no longer married, sibling relations may be more important for females since their contacts extend through out their lives. The black females are likely to renew their relationships with their siblings as they experience divorce and their husbands die.

The study also reveals that there is a negative relationship between visiting friends and life satisfaction for black females. As stated earlier, the frequency of interaction may not be as significant a factor in explaining life satisfaction as the quality of interaction. Qualitative variables should be included in future research to determine the influence of friendship contacts on the life satisfaction of black females.

The present findings suggest that the adjustment to aging with respect to life satisfaction may be different for black elderly males compared to females. Demographic, social, and familial variables have different impacts on the well-being of the sample across sex groups. The results of the study suggest that the adjustment-to-age models are quite different for black elderly males and females. The needs of black females are quite different from those of black males. The findings support earlier arguments that the black elderly should be treated as a heterogeneous group in formulating and designing social services programs. Before drawing broad generalizations about the patterns of adjustment of aging among blacks with no regard for sex difference, systematic research on familial, social, economic and psychological factors must be conducted in samples in the future with larger populations that are more representative of the black elderly.

REFERENCES

Allen, W. R. Class, culture, and family organization: The effects of class and race on family structure in urban America. *Journal of Comparative Family Studies,* 1979, *10,* 301-313.

Alston, J., Lowe, G., and Wrigley, A. Socioeconomic correlates of four dimensions of self-perceived satisfaction. *Human Organization,* 1972, *33,* 99-102.

Bild, B. and Havighurst, R. Senior citizens in great cities: The case of Chicago. *Gerontologist,* 1976, *16,* No. 1, part II.

Clemente, F., and Sauer, W. Race and morale of the urban aged. *Gerontologist,* 1974, *14,* 342-344.

Donnenwerth, G. V., Guy, R. F., and Norvell, M. J. Life satisfaction among older persons: Rural-urban and racial comparisons. *Social Science Quarterly,* 1978, *59,* 578-583.

Edwards, J. N., and Klemmack, D. L. Correlates of life satisfaction: A re-examination. *Journal of Marriage and the Family,* 1973, *35,* 51-57.

Hays, W. C., and Mindel, C. H. Extended kinship relations in black and white families. *Journal of Marriage and the Family,* 1973, *35,* 51-57.

Jackson, J. J. Negro aged: Toward needed research in social gerontology. *Gerontologist,* 1971, *11,* 52-57.

Jackson, J. J. Black aged in quest of the Phoenix. In *Triple Jeopardy-Myth or Reality.* Washington, DC: National council on the Aged, 1972.

Jackson, J. J. *Minorities and Aging.* Belmont, CA: Wadsworth Publishing Co.

Jackson, J. S., Bacon, J. D., and Peterson, J. Life satisfaction among Black urban elderly. *International Journal of Aging and Human Development,* 1977-78, *8,* 169-179.

Larson, R. Thirty years of research on the subjective wellbeing of older Americans. *Journal of Gerontology,* 1978, *33,* 109-125.

Markides, K. S., and Martin, H. W. A causal model of life satisfaction among the elderly. *Journal of Gerontology,* 1979, *34,* 36-93.

McAdoo, H. P. Factors related to stability in upwardly mobile black families. *Journal of Marriage and the Family,* 1978, *40,* 761-776.

Medley, M. L. Satisfaction with life among persons sixty-five years and older. *Journal of Gerontology,* 1976, *31,* 448-455.

Messer, M. Race differences in selected dimensions of the elderly. *Gerontologist,* 1968, *8,* 245-249.

Moore, J. W. Situational factors affecting minority aging. *The Gerontologist,* 1971, *11,* part II, 88-93.

National Urban League. *Double Jeopardy: The older Negro in America.* National Urban League, Washington, DC, 1964.

Neugarten, B., Havighurst, R., and Tobin, S. The measurement of life satisfaction. *Journal of Gerontology,* 1961, *16,* 134-143.

Palmore E., and Luikart, C. Health and social factors related to life satisfaction. *Journal of Health and Social Behavior,* 1972, *13,* 68-80.

Rao, V. N., and Rao, V. V. P. Life satisfaction in the black elderly: An exploratory study. *International Journal of Aging and Human Development,* 1982, 14.

Sauer, W. Morale of the urban aged: A regression analysis by race. *Journal of Gerontology,* 1977, *32,* 600-608.

Solomon, B. Social and protective services. *In Community services and the black elderly.* Andrus Gerontology Center, University of Southern California, Los Angeles, 1972.

Spreitzer, E., and Synder, E. Correlates of life satisfaction among the aged. *Journal of Gerontology,* 1974, *29,* 454-458.

Stack, C. B. *All Our Kin: Strategies for Survival in a Black Community,* Harper and Row, New York, 1974.

The Representation of Aging in Pop/Rock Music of the 1960s and '70s

Michael J. Leitner

ABSTRACT. The impact of pop/rock music on youth's attitudes toward aging is examined in this paper. Nine pop/rock songs from the 1960s and '70s with relevance to old age and aging were content analyzed. The aged are presented as sad and lonely beings in most of the songs analyzed. Further study in this area is recommended in order to examine the effects of pop/rock music on people's attitudes toward aging.

INTRODUCTION

The influence of various forms of media on attitudes toward aging has been the focus of several studies (Ansello, 1977; Peterson and Eden, 1977; Clarke, 1980; and Kubey, 1980). This study is concerned with the representation of old age and aging in the pop/rock music of the 1960s and '70s.

One purpose of this study is to examine the images of old age and aging presented in the pop/rock music of the 1960s and '70s, and the possible influence this might have on the attitudes toward aging of teenagers and young adults. Music is also examined in this paper as a means of exploring people's attitudes toward old age and aging.

REVIEW OF LITERATURE

Ansello (1977) examined the extent of age stereotyping in 656 children's books. Ansello concluded that the overall picture of older

---

Dr. Michael J. Leitner is Assistant Professor, Recreation Administration Dept., California State University, Chico, CA 95929. Dr. Leitner has MA and PhD degrees in Recreation, as well as Master's and Doctoral level certificates of concentration in Gerontology from the University of Maryland. Dr. Leitner has published several articles on the topic of recreation and aging and has produced a videotape, "Bridging the Gap," on the topic of intergenerational recreation activities.

persons presented in children's literature is that of relatively unimportant, unexciting, and unimaginative individuals. The author recognized the possible influence of children's literature on the attitudes of youth toward the elderly. Ansello recommended increased concern by educational gerontologists in this area.

A similar study by Peterson and Eden (1977) examined the images of older persons presented in 53 books for adolescents. According to the authors, the literature reviewed failed to present a positive image of the elderly, although it did not present negative portrayals of the aged either. Peterson and Eden discussed the importance of books and the media in shaping the attitudes of adolescents toward older persons. According to the authors, many adolescents have little contact with the aged; thus, the media and books influence the attitudes of adolescents toward older persons.

In contrast to Peterson's and Eden's study, Clark (1980) examined 120 poems written by 22 contemporary American poets age 60 and over for content related to aging. Clark found both positive and negative presentations of aging in the poetry he examined. Clark discussed the value of utilizing poetry in exploring one's feelings about aging.

Kubey (1980) reviewed studies on the elderly's image on television. According to Petersen (1973) and Aronoff (1974), the elderly are underrepresented on television. According to Aronoff, the image of aging on television is quite negative. Signorielli and Gerbner (1977) also stated that television shows present a negative image of old age.

In summary, the aforementioned literature was concerned with the influence of various forms of media on attitudes toward aging. The representation of aging in pop/rock music is an area of study which has thus far been neglected in the gerontological literature.

PROCEDURES

A collection of over 200 albums (containing over 2,000 songs) were reviewed for songs with relevance to old age and aging. Although this collection of albums by no means represents the universe of pop/rock music of the 1960s and '70s, the songs analyzed include those by some of the most popular and influential groups and individual artists of this time period (e.g., The Beatles, and Simon and Garfunkel).

Nine songs were selected for analysis. These songs were played for a college class titled "Recreation for the Aged" and were content analyzed as part of a pilot study. In the following section, excerpts and interpretations for each song are presented.

ANALYSIS OF SONGS

"Ding Dong, Ding Dong" by George Harrison is not really concerned with old age or aging, yet this song is an example of negative stereotyping of the aged. In the song, the phrases "Ring out the old, Ring in the new; Ring out the false, Ring in the true" are repeated several times. In this song, the word "old" clearly has a negative connotation. Thus, this song supports gerontologists' contentions that the words "old," "elderly," and "aged" have negative implications and that other terms should be used in their place to denote persons over age 65.

"Hello in There" by John Prine touches on the loneliness many of the elderly face. "Old trees just grow stronger; Old rivers grow wider every day; But old people, they just grow lonesome; Waitin' for someone to say; Hello in there." These phrases depict the irony of society's maltreatment of the aged: as things age in nature, they become more highly valued; conversely, in society, people become devalued as they grow into old age.

"When I'm Sixty-Four" by John Lennon and Paul McCartney (The Beatles) is one of the most well-known songs of the '60s related to old age. Although somewhat of a humorous, light-hearted love song, Lennon and McCartney also present stereotypes of the aged as decaying, sedentary beings. For example, the lines "When I get older, losing my hair; You can knit a sweater by the fireside; Doing the garden, digging the weeds, who could ask for more; and Yours sincerely, wasting away" are examples of phrases which elicit negative images of the aged.

"Father and Son" by Cat Stevens deals with the aging process through a dialogue between a father and son. A positive outlook on old age is set forth, particularly in the line "Look at me, I am old, but I'm happy." Contrary to many other songs and poems, this song about an old and young person portrays the older person as the happier individual.

"Treat Her Gently—Lonely Old People" by Paul McCartney presents an overwhelmingly depressing picture of old age. The lines "Here we sit, two lonely old people, eaking out lives away," and "Here we sit, out of breath, and nobody asked us to play—Old People's Home for the Day" obviously present old age as an unhappy time, marked by poor health and loneliness.

"Good Company" by Brian May (Queen) describes the life cycle through the eyes of an older person. "The work devoured my waking hours; Now I'm old, I puff my pipe, but no-one's there to see; I ponder on the lesson of my life's insanity." These lines depict the loneliness of old age, and reflect an older man's regrets for being too caught up in his work to really appreciate life.

"Voices of Old People" was recorded by Art Garfunkel in various locations, including several nursing homes; on the tape, segments of conversations with senior citizens can be heard, along with sounds of apparent pain and suffering. The voices taped seem to be of very old and frail persons. Because many adolescents have very limited exposure to elders, it is conceivable that "Voices of Old People" negatively influenced many teenagers' attitudes toward aging by portraying elders as frail and pathetic beings.

The next two selections on Simon and Garfunkel's *Bookends* album, "Old Friends," and "Bookends Theme," also deal with old age. "Old Friends" paints a vivid and tragic picture of being old and living in the city. The lines "How terribly strange to be seventy," and "Old friends, memory brushes the same years, silently sharing the same fear. . ." capture the pitifulness of old age which Simon and Garfunkel seem to be expressing. "Bookends Theme" seems to deal with the final stages of life in old age; the song begins with "Time it was" and ends with "Preserve your memories, they're all that's left you."

The songs selected for analysis in this paper present diverse representations of old age and aging. However, a theme common to most of the songs is that of loneliness and sadness in old age. While some of the interpretations presented in this paper may not represent what the authors of the songs actually intended, many of the songs analyzed elicit very clear messages about old age and aging.

DISCUSSION

Content analysis of pop/rock music can be a useful activity in exploring college students' attitudes toward aging. In addition to pop/rock music, it might also be interesting to examine the music of artists age sixty and over. Music-analysis activities can be conducted with senior citizens as well, in order to explore seniors' attitudes toward aging. In conducting such activities, it is desirable to use music appropriate for the group involved (e.g., some older persons might be unresponsive to pop/rock music).

It is difficult to estimate the amount of influence music has on the attitudes toward aging of teenagers and young adults. Regardless of the degree of influence music has on attitudes toward aging, it is apparent that pop/rock music of the 1960s and '70s has been an important influence on the lives of teenagers and young adults during the past two decades. Given this fact, it is important to examine the impact of pop/rock music on teenagers' and young adults' attitudes toward old age and aging. Further research in this area, including experimental study on this topic, might yield important information on the effects of pop/rock music on youth's attitudes toward aging the aged.

MUSIC SELECTIONS

Garfunkel, A. "Voices of Old People." *Bookends.* New York, NY: Columbia Records, 1967.

Harrison, G. "Ding Dong, Ding Dong." *Dark Horse.* New York, NY: Apple Records, Inc., 1974.

Lennon, J., and McCartney, P. "When I'm Sixty Four." *Sgt. Pepper's Lonely Hearts Club Band.* Hollywood, CA: Capitol Records, 1967.

May, B. "Good Company." *A Night at the Opera.* Los Angeles, CA: Warner Communications, Inc., 1975.

McCartney, P. "Treat Her Gently—Lonely Old People." *Venus and Mars.* New York, NY: McCartney Music, Inc., 1975.

Simon, P. "Bookends Theme." *Bookends.* New York, NY: Columbia Records, 1967.

———. "Old Friends." *Bookends.* New York, NY: Columbia Records.

Stevens, C. "Father and Son." *Tea For The Tillerman.* Hollywood, CA: A & M Records, 1970.

BIBLIOGRAPHY

Ansello, E. F. Age and ageism in children's first literature. *Educational Gerontology,* 1977, *2,* 255-74.

Aronoff, C. Old age in prime time. *Journal of Communication,* 1974, *24,* 86-87.

Clark, M. The poetry of aging: Views of old age in contemporary American poetry. *Gerontologist,* 1980, *20*(2), 88-91.

Kubey, R. W. Television and aging: Past, present, and future. *Gerontologist,* 1980, *20*(1), 16-35.

Petersen, M. The visibility and image of old people on television. *Journalism Quarterly,* 1973, *50,* 569-73.

Petersen, D. A., and Eden, D. Z. Teenagers and aging: Adolescent literature as an attitude source. *Educational Gerontology,* 1977, *2,* 311-25.

Signorielli, N., and Gerbner, G. The image of the elderly in prime-time television drama. *Generations,* 1978, *3,* 10-11.

Building Activities into a Network of Community-Based Supports

Barry Jay Glass

ABSTRACT. The Senior Citizens Health Center at St. Luke's Hospital was established in 1975 as an outpatient health facility for older adults. The clinic provides a range of services which support the clients in maintaining themselves in as independent a fashion as possible. This article enumerates a number of group activities that engage this clinic population; these activities are geared toward providing a network of continuing community support, and are integrated into a total package of health care delivery.

In 1975, St. Luke's Hospital, located in downtown Denver, opened its Senior Citizens Health Center. The Center now serves as an outpatient clinic for 2500 seniors over the age of 65; these seniors utilize the facilities of the hospital to receive their primary medical care. The hospital is in close proximity to two senior citizen highrises operated by the Denver Housing Authority. Additionally, the Capital Hill District, which lies south of the hospital, holds the largest concentration of senior citizens in the Denver Metropolitan Area. Transportation to and from the clinic, for those without ready access to private or public transportation, is provided by local community agencies, as well as an eight-passenger van with wheelchair lift; this van is shared by the clinic and the hospital blood bank. The van is also an integral part of the activity program of the clinic, for it provides the clients with access to services they would otherwise be unable to use.

The primary functioning of the clinic revolves around the delivery of health care services to our over 65 years of age population. We are staffed by six geriatric physicians whose practice is limited to working with our clinic patients. Additionally, we operate

Barry Jay Glass, MSSA is a Partner in *Aging Consultants and Trainers* (ACT) and a Social Worker and Program Planner at the Senior Citizens Health Center, Denver, Colorado.

55

with three geriatric nurse practitioners, a number of LPNs and RNs, a clinic manager, three clinic social workers, unit clerks, secretaries, and a variety of medical, nursing, and social work students. There are also a number of medical consultants who remain available to our clinic population. We have found the health care delivery system to be prime ground on which to build a total patient/client care plan. Through a variety of channels involving direct, indirect, and self-referral, a large number of clients become identified as "at risk" at one time or another. These clients, it is felt, could benefit from contact from one of the social workers. It is through this process of referral that clients begin to hook into a program of continued activity.

The continuity of care we provide for our patients is all important. If, for any reason, our patients require hospitalization, they are admitted to St. Luke's Hospital, and followed by their assigned clinic physician. If they are placed in a long-term care facility, their doctors make every attempt to continue to provide care. If the client is familiar to a clinic social worker, that social worker becomes the "team leader" for discharge planning. This social worker will continue to provide follow-up as needed, whether discharge be to a nursing home, or back to the community with home based supports.

The activity program of the clinic plays an integral part in supporting some clients who continue to live within the greater community. By offering a variety of programming, the clinic attempts to create a climate in which a community of self-support can begin and later flourish. By reminding the seniors of their own specialness, we are reinforcing their sense of self-worth and suggesting that they themselves are their own most valuable resource.

The programs we offer change as the need for services change. We as practitioners often shift interest and will explore alternative activities as our own levels of job intensity rise and fall. As facilitators, we are in fact members of a group we serve to help create and so must ourselves find the tasks and associations exciting, rewarding, and challenging. We may also find a group taking on a life of its own and be able to exist without our help and/or interference. If so, the better, for we are ultimately concerned with enhancing the seniors' abilities to help themselves. If they can build bridges with each other and create networks that exist outside of our group context, then we have indeed provided a useful service.

It must be noted that the activities to be described below are an essential part of a total health care plan. Their importance in the maintenance of functional abilities cannot be minimized. They are to be judged as on par with the work of our nurse practitioners, and yes, even our physicians. We must provide the very context of life so that orders of proper medication, diet, and exercise be followed. One must first want to live. Only then will there be motivation for pursuing optimal health care. For those seniors who find themselves isolated *against their wishes,* activities provide an important key to the re-opening of self.

The activities offered at the Senior Citizens Health Center of St. Luke's Hospital have included the following:

Women's Socialization Group. The members of this group are isolated women who continue to live in the community. They support each other in weekly activities, which aid to increase socialization skills. Our clinic van is used to provide transportation. Activities include holiday luncheons at members' homes, movies, trips to the Colorado mountains, excursions to Denver museums, parks, etc. The functional levels within the group vary, which adds to the sense of support as those who are more mobile help those who are not as mobile.

Men's Socialization Group. For the cohort of men who are now aged, retirement may have proved to be most devastating. Without the male companionship of fellow workmates, many gentlemen are isolated from each other. This loss of work role oftentimes leads to a sense of worthlessness. By providing men an opportunity to meet with each other, they are once again able to establish strong male associational ties. The group affords them the opportunity to rediscover their talents. A retired upholsterer, after boasting of his skills, began to craft chairs, cushions, and car seats for group and staff members alike. The activities of the men's group are similiar to those of the women's group. We often find the nature of the activity secondary to the opportunity it gives the men for getting together.

Water Exercise Group. A local YMCA has donated pool space so that our seniors who are arthritic and pre-arthritic can meet weekly to engage in this most beneficial of activities. We concentrate on simple stretching and range of motion exercises and stress the importance of gradual improvement and results. The water serves as a wonderful medium; it gives the participants an increased sense of mastery as they feel themselves moving in ways they have previously been unable to on land. The most difficult part of group organizing has been convincing the clients to come out of the locker rooms in their bathing suits, and in the case of an 84 year old woman, an athletic tee-shirt and gym shorts! The selfconsciousness soon disappears, and the group has a great time exercising, comparing notes, encouraging, and planning potluck luncheons (after a hard hour of exercise, what better reward).

Options for Wellness. A pot-pourri of client and instructor interest, this group is exposed to any number of topics related to self-help in health care. We exercise regularly, and include yoga, tai' chi', and dancercize in the program. We provide guest speakers from our own staff, i.e., nurse practitioners, to discuss nutrition, medication, heart disease, how to talk to your doctor, etc. Outside resources have been tapped to provide information concerning topics ranging from consumer protection to reflexology. The group offers their own suggestions and home remedies are shared and passed on. The group does not serve to replace the role of the physician; it, in fact, provides an adjunct to the doctor's recommendations. If we can teach someone that meditation for the purposes of stress reduction may assist in the lowering of blood pressure, then the client may feel more of a part of his/her own health care and more likely to stay on a plan which may include medication prescribed by a physician.

TLC Clinic. The association which links elders in the community with youngsters is oftentimes ignored. What better way to encourage feelings of self-worth than to allow an older person the opportunity to rediscover the joys of a young infant? Our hospital OB-GYN clinic is located next to our Senior clinic, and the nurses who helped with post-partum exams were hard pressed about the question of "What do we do about the baby?" And we said, "Why not let our patients hold the babies while the mothers undergo their exams?" We solicited donations of rocking chairs and toys and now have "grandmothers on duty" to help watch, feed, and change the babies. (We have yet to recruit any "grandfathers.") The women trade secrets, argue over mothering techniques, and most importantly, are given the chance to touch and be touched.

School Volunteer Program. Through a small mini-grant from the Colorado State Department of Education, we have been able to expand our interests in connecting the generations. We are bringing seniors into a local elementary school to act as aids and tutors. Additionally, we are identifying those seniors who are willing to share their specialness with children; these adults are offering their skill and their time to the school. An elderly artist is teaching finger painting to the children; two older Mexican-American sisters have cooked tortillas with the class; an older man who was one of the original Black Cowboys shares his experiences and brings in spurs and saddles for the children to see, touch, and feel. We also take the group on joint excursions, where we pair an older adult with a first grader. Together, they spend the time exploring the facility, i.e., an historical museum, and learn a bit about each other in the process. The grant we work under affords us the opportunity to demonstrate the need for such interaction by documenting our program with film and video. We also pay our "volunteers" a small fee for their time and materials. In addition, the teacher and clinic social worker build aging into the classroom curriculum so that the children may begin to discard some of the myths they may hold regarding "old people." We offer the experiences of our clients as a constant reminder that aging is individualized and can be continually meaningful.

Caregivers Support Group. In the Senior Citizens Health Center, we identified a number of women who were caring for husbands who were disabled: physically, mentally, or both. We tended to find more women caring for men, although we were able to learn of some men caring for disabled wives. These caregivers often feel isolated and hold feelings such as guilt and anger which they see as inappropriate to express. Additionally, these clients tend to neglect their own physical and mental health as they care for others. We found that these caregivers need a respite from their responsibilities and a chance to talk with each other about mutual concerns. By meeting regularly, this group has formed a network of community support and individual members have been able to identify their needs and seek ways to help themselves and others.

It is my belief that we are by nature social beings. Some older adults may choose to spend their lives alone and for these people, activity, for its own sake, may serve no useful purpose. In designing our activities and group programming, we seek to reach those who have not chosen their aloneness as a way of life, but have become isolated for any number of social, psychological, medical and/or economic reasons. The activities offered are only the vehicle with which we hope to connect these people with each other. As indicated earlier, *what* is done may sometimes be secondary to the fact that *something* is being done. If you can offer opportunity and interest, then your clients may feel the nourishment we all need in order to overcome fears of coming out and reaching out. By offering a comforting environment, we may attract those isolated elderly who have so much to give to us and each other. Additionally, we must not negate ourselves and our own interests in designing activities for our clients. By jointly pursuing mutual interests, activities that will generate can benefit all of us. Only then can we begin to interchange the roles of helper and helpee, and acknowledge that power lies in working together and not in controlling.

The programs described above are programs in a constant state of flux. They do not always run smoothly, and problems of logistics, staffing, and client participation are ever present. This article does not attempt to identify a model program of activity; it serves only to demonstrate a range of possibilities that can exist at one setting, and at one particular time. It also serves to support those of us who continue to work in the field of aging. We as helpers must continually justify our own wills to live as we work with a population who oftentimes needs our energy to help them with a daily struggle of survival. It is through this most important of connections that we engage together in the activity of being.

Musical Skill Level Self-Evaluation in Non-Institutionalized Elderly

Alicia Clair Gibbons

ABSTRACT. To determine if primarily Caucasian non-institutionalized elderly persons were satisfied with their musical skill levels, 13 male and 139 female subjects were asked to evaluate their current and their desired musical skill levels. The data indicated subjects generally desired an increase in their current musical skills. While 52 percent of the subjects who rated singing skills indicated a desire for better musical skills, 90 percent of the subjects who rated playing skills desired better ones. When general or overall musical skill was considered, 84 percent of the subjects indicated a desire for better skill. All results were highly statistically significant, $p < .001$.

The study indicates that the majority of Caucasian female non-institutionalized elderly persons in a limited population sample are not necessarily satisfied with current musical skill levels and would like to improve them. These results cannot be generalized to all elderly non-institutionalized persons, however, due to the restricted sample used in this study. Even so, it is possible that some elderly persons who are interested in music are also interested in improving their musical skills. Therefore, they may willingly participate in educational programs designed to improve musical skills. They may prefer such educational programs to those designed merely to maintain minimal or current musical skills levels.

INTRODUCTION

The number of persons over age 65 in the United States has increased from 4.1 percent of the population in 1900 to almost 11 percent in 1980. Based on that trend the projected population increase will reach an estimated 17 percent by the year 2020 (Siegel, 1976). One consequence of the growing population is the increased demand

61

by the elderly for programs and services which meet their various needs. As a result, federal and state policies and programs have attempted to meet those demands (Lawrence and Leeds, 1978).

Among elderly persons' demands are those for programs which increase life satisfaction and improve quality of life. Attempts to meet these demands have resulted in the development of many programs such as congregate meals, day care, and activity center programs. Observation of various programs reveals that music is pervasive in them. Further observation reveals, however, that musical activities often involve passive participation, such as music listening. Programs which include opportunities for more active music participation usually require minimal musical skills. Because of the minimal requirements those skills are often ones acquired at an earlier age, even as early as childhood.

Such minimal skill requirements in music activities may reflect the biases of program planners. These planners may tend to have low expectations for the elderly in music activities. Planners may assume elderly persons cannot or do not want to develop musical skills. These biases, and other biases related to musical skill development in the elderly, are necessarily based on intuition and limited experience. Reliance on intuition and experience is understandable because musical characteristics of elderly persons are relatively unknown. A review of the literature reveals a paucity of research concerning musical characteristics of elderly persons. Knowledge of those characteristics is imperative in the design and implementation of appropriate music program activities for the elderly.

One aspect of elderly persons' musical characteristics is their preference for musical skill level development or lack of development. Information concerning whether elderly persons prefer to increase or not to increase their musical skill levels seems prerequisite to appropriate music programming. Without such information most program planners will exclude developmental opportunities in music while elderly persons may prefer the developmental activities to mere maintenance activities.

The purpose of this study was to determine if elderly persons in a limited population sample were satisfied with their current musical skills or if they preferred to develop better ones. The determination was derived from comparisons of subjects' self-evaluations of current musical skills with their indicated desire for musical skills.

METHOD

Subjects

Subjects were participants in the federally subsidized congregate meal program at 15 sites in rural and urban areas of Kansas, Missouri, and California. Sites were chosen to represent diverse socioeconomic backgrounds. Program participants, age 65 years or older, were asked to volunteer for the project when a research proposal was presented at the sites. Subjects were told they could discontinue their participation in the project at any time. The original sample included 189 subjects; however, due to drop out only 152 completed the project. Of them, 13 were males and 139 were females. Two of the female subjects were black, one subject was American Indian, and all other subjects were Caucasian.

Procedure

Subjects were asked to rate (A) how "good" they currently were at music; and (B) how "good" they would like to be at music according to the following categories: not good, so-so, good, and very good. Subjects were then asked to judge their current singing skills and their current playing skills by marking all applicable items in a list of 10 skill level descriptors. The descriptors were placed on a continuum for singing and playing. The continuum for singing ranged from "cannot carry a tune" to "currently sing or have sung professionally"; and the continuum for playing ranged from "cannot play at all" to "currently play or have played professionally." A score of one point was assigned to each skill level descriptor and a total additive score was computed for each subject's singing skills and for each subject's playing skills.

Subjects participated in the project in groups of 20 or less for the amount of time necessary for all to complete the tasks. Each subject was required to read items in large print and circle responses. All subjects indicated they understood the tasks and proceeded independently.

Content validity was established by three experts through an item validation procedure. The Kendall Coefficient of Concordance W (Daniel, 1978) was computed for agreement among the experts. Reliability was established through a test-retest procedure with 11 subjects whose data were not included in the experimental study. A Pearson correlation coefficient was computed between the test and the retest responses for each item.

RESULTS

The content validation procedure yielded a Kendall Coefficient of Concordance W of .95, $p < .01$. The items were considered valid. All Pearson correlations computed in the reliability study fell in a range from .95 to 1.00 and all were significant, $p < .05$. The items were accepted as reliable.

Because normal distribution assumptions were not met, the experimental data were treated with the contingency table of cross-tabulation analysis and the chi square test was used to test significance (Nie, Hull, Jenkins, Steinbrenner, and Bent, 1975).

Table 1 shows the crosstabulated ratings of desired musical skills by ratings of current overall musical skills. Only 24 of 150 subjects who responded did not indicate a desire for better overall musical skills. Those 24 subjects were considered satisfied with their current skill levels. The remaining 126 subjects, or 84 percent, desired

TABLE 1

Crosstabulated Ratings of Desired Musical Skill by
Ratings of Current Overall Musical Skill

Judgment of Musical Skill	Not good No music activity	So-So	Good	Very Good	Row Total
Desired Musical Skill					
Not good	0	2	0	0	2
So-So	12	10	0	0	22
Good	21	45	7	0	73
Very good	5	22	21	5	53
Column Total	38	79	28	5	150

better musical skills which indicates they were not satisfied with their current skill levels. The chi square test for the difference between observed and expected numbers of subjects who desired better musical skills was highly significant, $p < .001$. That is, there was a significant number of persons who desired better overall musical skills than they already had.

The results of the crosstabulated ratings of desired musical skills by ratings of current singing skills are presented in Table 2. Seventy-two subjects indicated they had no desire to improve musical skills because they rated their desired skill levels equal to or less than their ratings for current skills. However, 80 subjects, or 53 percent of the sample who rated themselves at various singing skill levels, indicated a desire for better musical skills. The chi squared test for observed and expected numbers of subjects who desired better musical skills was highly significant, $p < .001$. The results indicate that some elderly preferred better singing skills than they had; therefore, they were not satisfied with their current singing skill levels.

Table 3 displays the crosstabulation computed for ratings of desired musical skill by ratings of current playing skills. The results show 132 of 147 subjects who responded, or 90 percent of the sample, desired an increase in playing skills. The chi square test for differences between observed and expected numbers of subjects who desired better playing skills was highly significant, $p < .001$. Those data show subjects preferred better playing skills than they currently had which indicated their dissatisfaction with their current skills.

DISCUSSION

Even though this study was conducted in congregate meal sites in which participants were representative of an elderly non-institutionalized population, volunteers for the study were primarily Caucasian females. Elderly males and persons of races other than Caucasian generally did not participate. Among others several possible explanations for their nonparticipation include: lack of interest, apprehension, and tendencies to drop out.

Because of the large number of female subjects, the research sample was restricted and did not represent a normal distribution of non-institutionalized persons throughout the population. Consequently, any interpretation of results must reflect the population

TABLE 2

Crosstablulated Ratings of Desired Musical
Skill by Ratings of Current Singing Skill

Singing Ability	Not good	So-So	Good	Very Good	Row Total
Desired Musical Skill					
Not good	1	1	1	0	3
So-So	5	13	4	0	22
Good	7	34	20	13	74
Very good	2	21	11	19	53
Column Total	15	69	36	32	152

TABLE 3

Crosstabulated Ratings of Desired Musical Skill by
Ratings of Current Playing Skill

Playing Ability	No good Never played	So-So	Good	Very Good	Row Total
Desired Musical Skill					
Not Good	3	0	0	0	3
So-So	16	4	1	0	21
Good	34	31	3	2	70
Very Good	12	25	12	4	53
Column Total	65	60	16	6	147

sample restrictions and generalizations to all persons in an elderly population are not possible.

The data indicate that a majority of non-institutionalized elderly Caucasian female subjects generally desired an increase in musical skills. While 52 percent of the subjects who rated singing skills indicated a desire for better musical skills, 90 percent of the subjects who rated playing skills desired better skills. When general or overall musical skill was considered, 84 percent of the subjects indicated a desire for better skills. Implications are that a majority of non-institutionalized elderly Caucasian females are not satisfied with their current levels of musical skills and would like better ones.

These results refute the assumption that elderly Caucasian women are satisfied with current musical skill levels. Elderly subjects in this limited sample preferred to have better musical skills to their current skill levels. As a result, programs for elderly should include opportunities to develop musical skills. Such developmental or educational programs may contribute more to some elderly Caucasian female persons' satisfaction than programs designed merely to maintain skills. Such satisfaction may result in preferences for educational programs over maintenance programs. Future research should explore such satisfaction and preference possibilities. Additional research might determine whether satisfaction from musical experiences in either developmental or maintenance programs contributes to improved quality of life.

REFERENCES

Birren, J. E., & Clayton, V. History of gerontology. In D. Woodruff & J. Birren (Eds.), *Aging*. New York: Van Nostrand, 1975.

Daniel, W. *Applied nonparametric statistics*. Boston: Houghton Mifflin Company, 1978.

Lawrence, W., & Leeds, S. *An inventory of federal income transfer programs*. White Plains, New York: Institute for Sociometric Studies, 1978.

Nie, N., Hull, C., Jenkins, J., Steinbrenner, K., & Bent, D. (2nd ed.) *Statistical package for the social sciences*. New York: McGraw-Hill Book Company, 1975.

Siegel, J. S. *Demographic aspects of aging and the older population in the United States* (Report No. 59). Special Studies Series P-23, Washington, D.C.: U.S. Department of Commerce, Bureau of the Census, U.S. Government Printing Office, May, 1976.

Physical Fitness and Self-Sufficiency in Persons Over 60 Years

Kay Flatten

ABSTRACT. The physical fitness factors of flexibility and muscular strength are discussed with respect to people over 60 years of age. Changes in joint ranges of motion and maximal muscular strength occurring with increasing age are presented. The relevance of these changes to activities of daily living and the maintenance of an independent lifestyle are the major theme of this article.

INTRODUCTION

Physical fitness is considered to include the biological functioning of muscles producing torque, of joint actions executing range of motion, and of cardiovascular efficiency in transporting oxygen to the body. Of these three fitness components, flexibility and strength are of primary importance in the basic performance of activities of daily living (ADLs). Independence and self-sufficiency in old age require that the individual be able to execute ADLs without assistance; therefore, the role of flexibility and strength in the maintenance of essential movements in older people is the subject of this article.

FLEXIBILITY

Range of motion (ROM) is the arc of active motion in a joint with the normal limits reported in degrees. Actions essential to lifting and moving the body include ankle dorsiflexion and plantarflexion, knee

Dr. Kay Flatten, PED is Assistant Professor of Kinesiology at Iowa State University, 246 P.E.B., Ames, Iowa 50011.

This article is the modified version of a paper presented at the Gerontology Workshop on Physical Activity and Aging, Iowa State University, Ames, Iowa, February 2, 1982. Research projects reported were sponsored by the Iowa State University Research Institute for Studies in Education and a Biomedical Research Support Grant from the National Institutes of Health Grant PHS/NIH grant no. 2 S07 RR07034-15.

flexion, hip flexion and extension. Motions requiring lifting and reaching for objects need ROM in shoulder and elbow flexion, also extension of the shoulder is useful in dressing. Figure 1 shows range of motion measures taken on the knee joint, and Figure 2 shows this

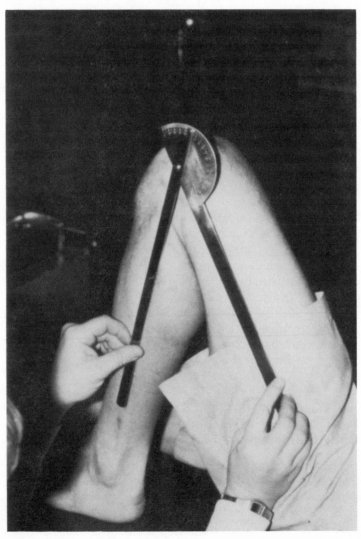

FIGURE 1. Range of motion for knee flexion is measured by a physical therapist (photograph by Darlene Paysen)

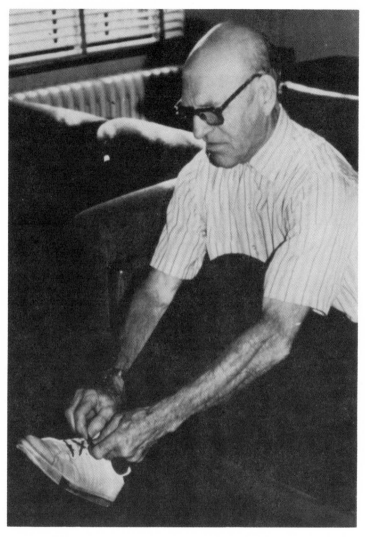

FIGURE 2. Range of motion for knee flexion is used while tying shoes (photograph by Darlene Paysen)

motion used in tying a shoe. The two essential questions for older populations is whether flexibility decreases significantly in healthy joints with advancing age, and how much ROM is required to accomplish the most important ADLs.

Until recently studies on changes in flexibility during aging have centered upon age ranges from childhood to maturity. In 1979 Boone and Azen measured 109 males from eighteen months to fifty-four years old. More recently, this author extended the age range from thirty to ninety years using 140 subjects. Both cross-sectional research designs revealed a decline in the normal limits of joint motion (see Table 1).

The loss of degrees of motion is of concern if the remaining mobility is insufficient for required ADLs. These demands have been studied for hip and knee motion (Johnston & Smidt, 1970; Laubenthal, Keyron, Smidt & Kettelkamp, 1972). The hip flexion needed for many common motions can be found in Figure 3. Hip ROM for seventy to ninety year old males and females plus and minus one standard deviation is represented by the shaded area. The

Table 1

Average Ranges of Motion* for Men and Women
in Three Adult Age Groups
From 30-95

Joint Motion	AGE N/Sex	30-59		60-69		70-95	
		5/M	35/F	18/M	33/F	16/M	34/F
ankle fl. (dorsi)		14.20	10.34	10.67	8.12	7.78	5.37
ankle ex. (plantar)		55.30	65.27	54.22	61.88	50.41	55.18
knee fl.		146.4	146.34	141.89	142.75	141.44	138.22
knee ex.		0.0	0.0	0.0	-.27	-.25	-.46
hip fl.		127	130.61	118.39	121.30	119.20	121.15
hip ex.		19.10	20.0	11.25	15.06	9.43	13.25
shoulder fl.		164.8	165.14	160.67	160.77	156.06	160.47
shoulder ex.		54.20	57.43	49.53	54.19	48.25	49.72
elbow fl.		150.90	152.50	143.83	150.05	146.34	150.53
elbow ex.		0.0	0.0	-.28	-.02	0.0	0.0
great toe ex.		66.00	77.46	67.50	71.69	67.66	65.63
cervical fl.		57.20	51.11	40.89	47.72	35.94	42.18
cervical ex.		68.80	66.46	50.39	58.50	54.75	53.59

* Values for ranges of motion are reported in degrees from the anatomical $0°$ position as outlined by the American Academy of Orthopaedic Surgeons.

solid bars coincide with the amount of hip flexion (+ and − one S.D.) used by adult males as reported by Johnston and Smidt (1970). These results seem to indicate that the only motions affected by decreasing flexibility would be squatting and for some people, stooping. The majority of the group maintained enough mobility to perform all the tasks without modification due to joint tightness.

Similar results were found for knee motions. This author found the mean ROM for seventy year olds and older in knee flexion to be 139°. Laubenthal, Smidt and Kettelkamp (1972) found the following knee motion requirements: stairs 83°, sitting 90°, tying shoes 105°, stooping 65°, and squatting 115°. Apparently, all motions would be possible for older people free from injured or diseased joints.

MUSCULAR STRENGTH

Muscular strength is a second fitness factor which has been studied in older populations. There are four classifications of strength evaluations. These are maximal isometric, isometric endurance, maximal isokinetic, and isokinetic endurance. Isometric contractions are static contractions at fixed limb positions. Isokinetic contractions are dynamic and measure strength throughout the full range of motion. Larsson's (1979) pioneer work in the area of strength at all ages has shown that maximal isometric and dynamic strength decrease after sixty years of age; however, endurance strength is not lost and in fact increases with age.

Maximal isokinetic strength is the element of greatest importance in retaining the capability to accomplish ADLs independently. This author studied maximal isokinetic strength in 65 males and females in the motions of knee flexion and extension, and dorsi plus plantarflexion of the ankle. In Figure 4 the muscular strengths of knee flexion and extension are recorded by a dynamometer and Figure 5 shows this strength being used in raising the weight of the body plus an object. Figure 6 shows the means for maximal isokinetic strength at $\pi/6$ radians/sec. for both sexes and age groups, where young adults were defined as thirty to fifty-nine and old adults were sixty to eighty-nine years of age.

All of the muscle groups tested were significantly stronger in males ($p < .01$) and all muscle groups except those producing ankle dorsiflexion were stronger in the younger adults ($p < .01$). Findings on the quadricep muscle group showed that young females were

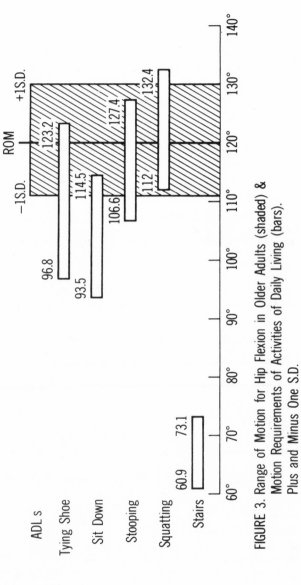

FIGURE 3. Range of Motion for Hip Flexion in Older Adults (shaded) & Motion Requirements of Activities of Daily Living (bars). Plus and Minus One S.D.

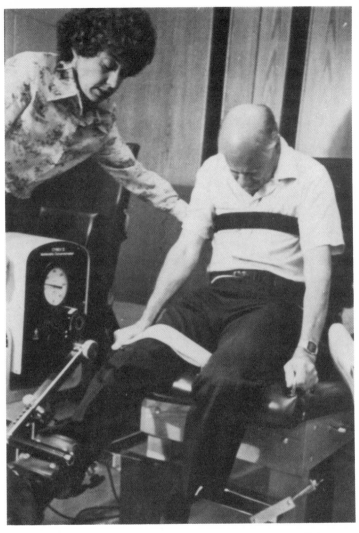

FIGURE 4. Maximal strength in knee extension is measured on a Cybex II dynamometer (photograph by Richard Trump)

78% as strong as young males while old females were only 64% as strong as old males. Older males were 77% as strong as younger males, while older females were only 64% as strong as their younger counterparts. Thus, females lost 36% of their strength with

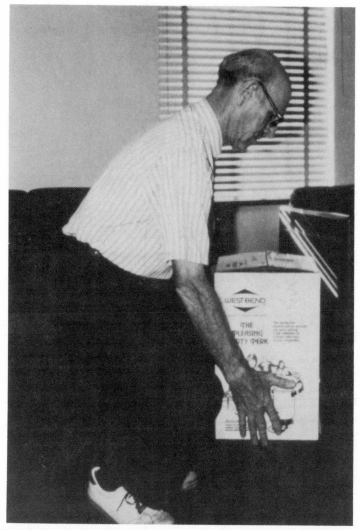

FIGURE 5. Muscular strength in knee extension is used while lifting the body's weight plus an object (photograph by Darlene Paysen)

age while males only lost 23%. Since females are weaker than males initially, this loss with age may have a greater effect on their execution of independent movement.

The question of how these strength results apply to daily life necessitates knowing how much torque is required to execute ADLs. Richards and Burke (1980) found that rising from a chair reproduced 80% of the observed maximal electrical activity of the quadricep muscles. This author analyzed a 52 kilogram (115 lb.) woman rising from a chair. The maximal mechanical torque at the knee joint required to lift her weight was 13 Nm per leg. A knee angle of 82° was present when the greatest torque was required from the quadricep muscles. The mean maximal torque value for that muscle group at an angle of 82° for 130 contractions by women over sixty was 23 Nm with a standard deviation of 15 Nm. This shows great variability and many first attempts only produced five to ten Nm with some women never getting more torque than this on

FIGURE 6. Isokinetic Strength in Two Adult Age Groups

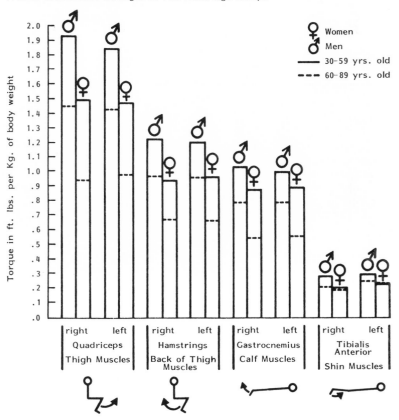

subsequent attempts. Any woman weighing more than 52 kg would require more torque than 13 Nm or else modify her motion. Modifications could include using arms to push, or rocking the trunk to build momentum.

If women lose 36% of their strength capacity and if 80% of their youthful capacity is required to rise from a chair, then there are probably many women over sixty who do modify the mechanics of rising from a chair. Since men have such a greater strength capacity at all ages than women they may not approach this crisis as soon as women. This is even more likely when the life expectancy of the two sexes is considered.

CONCLUSION

In conclusion, it is apparent that flexibility or range of motion declines with age but does not seem to endanger normal activity. On the other hand, strength declines in old age are significant enough to endanger ADLs, especially in females.

REFERENCES

Boone, Donna C., and Azen, Stanley P. Normal range of motion of joints in male subjects. *The Journal of Bone and Joint Surgery,* July 1979, *41*(5), pp. 756-759.

Johnston, Richard C., and Smidt, Gary L. Hip motion measurements for selected activities of daily living. *Clinical Orthopaedics and Related Research,* September-October 1970, Number 72, pp. 205-215.

Larsson, Lars, Grimby, Gunnar, and Karlsson, Jan. Muscle strength and speed of movement in relation to age and muscle morphology. *Respiratory Environment and Exercise Physiology,* January-March 1979, *43,* pp. 451-455.

Laubenthal, Keyron N., Smidt, Gary L., and Kettelkamp, Donald B. A quantitative analysis of knee motion during activities of daily living. *Physical Therapy,* January 1972, *52*(1), pp. 34-42.

Richards, Carol L., and Burke, D. L. Electromyographic activity in the quadriceps during isokinetic movements and locomotion after meniscal surgery. *Human Locomotion I: Pathological Gait to the Elite Athlete,* Biomechanics, London, Ontario, Canada, October 1980, pp. 76-77.

Levels of Senior Centers:
A Broadened View
of Group-Based Programs
for the Elderly

Penny A. Ralston

ABSTRACT. Using the National Institute of Senior Centers definition (NISC, 1978) as a basis, this paper presents a three-level classification of senior center programs, and tests the classification using statewide data collected in Iowa. The study focused on three aspects of the classification: (a) activities and services, (b) staffing and scheduling patterns, and (c) funding sources. Questionnaires were administered to 264 senior center directors and program leaders in Iowa. The findings lend support to the senior center classification, especially in terms of activities and services (exclusive versus inclusive) and staffing and scheduling patterns. In particular, the results suggest that senior clubs and congregate meals sites are providing many of the same supportive services as the traditional multipurpose senior center.

Research related to senior centers primarily has dealt with program development (Hoppa and Roberts, 1974; Jones, 1976; Pierce, 1975) and utilization (Demko, 1979; Downing, 1957; Hanssen et al., 1978; Kutner, Fanshel, Togo & Langner, 1956; Louis Harris & Associates, 1975; Rosow, 1967, Tissue, 1971). With the exception of Taietz (1976), who investigated voluntary organization and social agency conceptual models of the senior center, few studies have

Penny A. Ralston, PhD, is Assistant Professor, Department of Home Economics Education, Iowa State University, 222C MacKay Hall, Ames, IA 50011.

This study was supported in part by a 1979 Research Fellowship from the Gerontological Society of America. Appreciation is extended to the Iowa Commission on the Aging for support and guidance during this project.

been concerned with developing and/or testing models of senior center programs.

There is a great need for research in this area. First, there has not been a general consensus of what a senior center is. Early definitions such as that proposed by Frankel (1967) emphasized that a senior center should have a physical facility, regular scheduling of activities, paid staff, and definite funding sources. The recent definition developed by the National Institute of Senior Centers (NISC, 1978) has more global applications:

> A senior center is a community focal point on aging where older people as individuals or in groups come together for services and activities which enhance their dignity, support their independence and encourage their involvement in and with the community. (p. 15)

This expanded definition could prove useful in investigating various models of senior center programs.

In addition to the need for a better understanding of what a senior center is, there also is a need to determine the utility of senior centers as community "focal points." According to recent amendments to the Older Americans Act, senior centers are suggested as possible focal points for comprehensive service delivery. Whether the traditional senior center or perhaps less structured senior program models best meet the need for community focal points is still a question to be answered.

With the current legislation considering senior centers as possible focal points and with the paucity of research testing senior center definitions and models, it seems important to investigate the concept of the senior center. Thus, using the NISC definition of a senior center, this paper explores a framework for investigating a broadened view of these programs, and tests this framework using statewide data collected in Iowa.

Specifically, the objectives of this research were to:

1. Develop a classification of senior center programs using the NISC definition as a basis.
2. Test the validity of the senior center classification by using statewide Iowa data related to the areas of (a) activities and services, (b) staffing and scheduling patterns, and (c) funding sources.

CLASSIFICATION OF SENIOR CENTER PROGRAMS

Table 1 gives a detailed description of the classification of senior center programs in the study. The classification was developed by using available literature on senior centers (AOA, 1977; Task Force on Senior Center Development, 1978) and by acquiring the judgments of practitioners and policy-makers at the Iowa Commission on the Aging who had contact with group-based programs for the elderly. The classification is composed of three levels of senior center programs. Level One senior center programs are senior clubs or groups; Level Two programs are nutrition or congregate meal

Table 1

Classification of Senior Center Programs

Level One A club or group of older people that meets once or twice a month. The group has no permanent meeting place, but may rent or borrow a facility such as a church or community center. Programs offered are exclusive in nature, centering around social and recreational activities. Leadership within the club or group depends on volunteers as officers, and operational funds usually come from contributions or dues. Mainly due to the lack of funding and a permanent facility, the group may not be able to plan for additional activities or services.

Level Two A congregate meal site that is open several days (at least three) a week, with time reserved for more than just serving the meal (three or more hours). Although there is no permanent facility, the meal program may have a designated site for a period of a year or longer. Programs offered are exclusive in nature, with the meal being the primary activity. However, other activities and services are provided. Leadership at the nutrition site comes from paid staff (site manager) and volunteers. Title III-C of the Older Americans Act is the main funding source, although other funds can be generated. Due to the reliability of funding source, leadership, and the permanence of a facility, this level of program may be able to plan for additional activities and services.

Level Three A program that has a permanent facility specifically designed for older people, and is open several days (at least five) a week for a number of hours (5 or more). Because the facility is designed for older people and due to the number of hours open, the program has a flexible, drop-in environment. Programs offered are inclusive in nature, with a variety of activities (social, recreational, educational) and services provided. Leadership may come from both paid staff and volunteers. Funds are derived from a variety of local, state and federal sources. Due to the leadership, diverse nature of funding sources, permanence of a facility, and "drop-in" atmosphere, this level of program may already be multi-purpose. However, if that goal has not been reached, the program has the potential of offering an array of additional activities and services. This level also includes senior programs offered in community centers at least five days a week for six or more hours.

sites primarily funded by Title III of the Older Americans Act; and Level Three programs are traditional multi-purpose senior centers.

The levels differ due to two factors: (a) nature of current programming (inclusive versus exclusive) and (b) potential for additional programming. In terms of current programming, the levels ranged from exclusive programming (Level One) where only one or two services or activities are offered to inclusive programming (Level Three) where several services or activities are offered. Potential for future programming is based on the program's ability to expand in its range of services and activities. Again, this ranged from very limited ability to expand (Level One) to a great potential to expand (Level Three). Both nature of current programming and potential for additional programming depend upon type of facilities, staffing and scheduling capabilities, and funding sources.

Each of the levels within the classification could fit the NISC definition of a senior center. This is important because the NISC definition serves as the underlying criterion for the three levels in the classification. While the three levels may not represent the traditional view of the senior center, each has the potential of fulfilling the need for such a program in a particular community. This argument is supported by the Task Force for Senior Center Development commissioned by the Administration on Aging (Note 1). In a discussion of the similarity between nutrition sites and senior centers, the Task Force Report states: "many nutrition sites have programs which are similar in nature to senior center programs, offering a wide variety of recreational and social services in conjunction with the service of meals. Many nutrition sites consider themselves as senior centers" (p. 3). And in discussing social clubs for the aged, the report suggests that "club activities are often closely linked to other more formal community group-based service programs. Thus, the participation by older persons in club activities can serve as a bridge to other social service programs in time of need"(p. 3).

The present study was concerned with testing one main aspect of the senior center classification: nature of current programming. To test this aspect, the areas of activities and services, staffing and scheduling patterns, and funding sources were investigated. Data for the study were collected as a part of a larger effort to identify senior center programs in Iowa (Ralston, Note 2). Because of the emphasis on identification of programs, the study did not address (a) potential for future programming or (b) the types of facilities used in senior center programs. These aspects of the classification will need to be investigated in subsequent research.

DATA COLLECTION PROCEDURES

In order to test the classification of senior centers previously discussed, a survey questionnaire was administered to senior center directors and other program leaders in Iowa. The questionnaire included checklist-type questions related to activities and services, scheduling and staffing patterns, and funding sources. The instrument also included background information concerning the senior center director or program leader.

To reach as many programs as possible, the questionnaire was first sent to directors of the 13 area agencies on aging in Iowa. Using the list of programs at their disposal, the area agency directors forwarded copies of the questionnaire to senior programs in their respective areas. The letter accompanying the questionnaire stressed that leaders of a wide variety of senior programs should respond, not just those involved in programs traditionally considered senior centers.

Data from 264 usable questionnaires were used in the descriptive analysis for the study. The survey included 105 Level One programs, 70 Level Two programs and 89 Level Three programs. While Level One and Three programs were being identified for the first time, the number of Level Two programs represented 29% of the congregate meal programs in the state.

Because of the data collection procedures used, there were limitations in determining the response rate or the percentage of senior center directors/program leaders in Iowa that responded to the study. However, with the exception of a four-county area in the northeast corner of the state, the sample was representative of the geographical areas in Iowa (Ralston, Note 2). In addition, the sample reflected the proportion of rural/urban areas in Iowa with 44.7% of the returned questionnaires from communities with populations of less than 1,000, 38.2% from communities of 1,000 to 9,999, 5.7% from communities of 10,000 to 49,999, and 11.4% from communities with populations of 50,000 and over.

RESULTS

Activities and Services

The activities and services investigated in this study included (a) drop-in facilities, (b) recreation/leisure, (c) information and referral, (d) transportation, (e) escort, (f) health, (g) education, (h) outreach, and (i) congregate meals.[3]

Table 2

Frequencies and Percentages of Activities and
Services in Senior Centers
by Level of Program[a]

n=264

Activity or Service	Level of Program			Total Sample
	Level One	Level Two	Level Three	
Drop-in Facilities	10 (3.8)	27 (10.2)	79 (29.9)	116 (43.9)
Recreation/leisure	75 (28.4)	57 (21.6)	86 (32.6)	218 (82.6)
Information and Referral	35 (13.3)	41 (15.5)	58 (22.0)	134 (50.8)
Transportation	21 (8.0)	41 (15.5)	54 (20.5)	116 (43.9)
Escort	6 (2.3)	12 (4.5)	26 (9.8)	44 (16.7)
Health	10 (3.8)	37 (14.0)	51 (19.3)	98 (37.1)
Education	12 (4.5)	36 (13.6)	54 (20.5)	102 (38.6)
Outreach	31 (11.7)	41 (15.5)	48 (18.2)	120 (45.5)
Congregate Meals	9 (3.4)	60 (22.7)	56 (21.2)	125 (47.3)
Other Programs	35 (13.3)	8 (3.0)	39 (14.8)	82 (31.1)

[a]Percentages are in parentheses

Table 2 shows the frequencies and percentages for activities and services by level of senior center program. With the exception of recreation and congregate meal programs, the frequencies progressively increased from Level One through Level Three. The frequencies for recreation were higher at Level One than at Level Two, but rose again at Level Three. This finding was expected because Level One senior center programs are primarily recreational. The frequencies for congregate meal programs were higher at Level Two than at either Level One or Level Three. Again, this finding was expected because Level Two senior center programs have congregate meals as a main service.

Staffing and Scheduling Patterns

Staffing patterns were investigated by determining whether or not senior centers had (a) full-time directors, (b) paid staff, (c) volunteer staff, (d) policy boards, and (e) advisory committees. Scheduling patterns were determined by calculating the mean number of days and hours senior centers were open.

Table 3 shows the frequencies and percentages for staffing by level of program. Level Two and Three senior centers appear to have full-time directors, paid staff, policy boards and advisory committees much more frequently than Level One programs. The frequencies for volunteer staff were consistently high for all three levels of senior centers. Nutrition site councils, common to Level Two programs, were more often considered advisory committees than policy making boards.

In terms of scheduling, the days and hours a senior center was open tended to increase as the level of program increased. Level One programs were not included in calculating mean scores because most of these programs met once or twice a month for an undetermined number of hours. Level Two programs were open 3.4 days

Table 3

Frequencies and Percentages for Staffing
in Senior Centers by Level of Program [a]

n=264

Staffing	Level One	Level Two	Level Three	Total Sample
		Level of Program		
Senior Center Director (full-time)	7 (2.7)	43 (16.3)	50 (18.9)	100 (37.9)
Paid Staff	2 (0.8)	54 (20.5)	55 (20.8)	111 (42.0)
Volunteer Staff	25 (9.1)	51 (19.3)	72 (27.3)	147 (55.7)
Policy Board	9 (3.4)	15 (5.7)	44 (16.7)	68 (25.8)
Advisory Committee	17 (6.4)	52 (19.7)	63 (23.9)	132 (50.0)

[a]Percentages are in parentheses

per week for an average of 5.5. hours, while Level Three programs were open 5.3 days per week for 7.4 hours.

FUNDING SOURCES

The funding sources investigated in this study included: (a) Older Americans Act (OAA) social services, (b) OAA nutrition, (c) OAA senior centers, (d) state funds, (e) county and/or city funds, (f) Revenue Sharing, and (g) contributions and/or dues. The first three funding sources listed refer to Title III appropriations from the Older Americans Act.[4]

As shown in Table 4, Level Three senior centers received support primarily from contributions and/or dues, county-city funds and OAA nutrition funds, while Level Two programs were mostly fi-

Table 4

Frequencies and Percentages of Funding Sources
for Senior Centers by Level of Program[a]

n=264

Funding Source	Level of Program			Total Sample
	Level One	Level Two	Level Three	
OAA Social Services	2 (0.8)	36 (13.6)	29 (11.0)	67 (25.4)
OAA Nutrition	1 (0.4)	65 (24.6)	50 (18.9)	116 (43.9)
OAA Senior Center	2 (0.8)	7 (2.7)	21 (8.0)	30 (11.4)
State Funds	3 (1.1)	19 (7.2)	18 (6.8)	40 (15.2)
County or City Funds	7 (2.7)	28 (10.6)	57 (21.6)	92 (34.8)
Revenue Sharing	14 (5.3)	25 (9.5)	39 (14.8)	78 (29.5)
Contributions and/or Dues	76 (28.8)	37 (14.0)	68 (25.8)	181 (68.6)
Other	14 (5.3)	18 (6.8)	36 (13.6)	68 (25.8)

[a]Percentages are in parentheses

nanced through OAA nutrition funds, contributions and/or dues and OAA social services. Level One programs overwhelmingly were funded by contributions and/or dues.

Overall, contributions and dues was the most utilized funding source (68.6%) followed by OAA nutrition appropriations (43.9%) and county/city funds (34.8%). Funding sources most frequently listed in the "other" category included fund raising (e.g., craft and bake sales, raffles) and the United Way.

DISCUSSION AND IMPLICATIONS

The results of the study lend support to the senior center classification presented in this paper. Specifically, the results validate the exclusive/inclusive aspect of programming within the classification. In addition, the results suggest that staffing and scheduling patterns and funding sources are important factors in determining levels of senior center programs.

The findings supported the classification in terms of nature of current programming. In the classification, programming ranged from exclusive to inclusive as the level of program increased. The results showed this to be true, with the number of activities and services increasing as the level of program increased. Level One programs were, as expected, primarily recreational. Level Two programs had the highest frequencies for congregate meals, but also had other activities and services. This demonstrated the diversity of offerings within congregate meal programs, and showed their potential to serve elderly in a variety of ways. Level Three programs had the highest frequencies for all activities and services, suggesting that "traditional" senior centers also are providing a variety of activities and services to their consumers.

The results further validate the classification in terms of staffing and scheduling patterns. The classification suggested that as the level of program increased, the number of staff utilized and the accessibility (number of days and hours the program was open) also would increase. In terms of staffing, the results showed that both Level Two and Three programs had higher frequencies than Level One programs for full-time directors, paid staff and volunteer staff. As expected, Level One programs had lower frequencies for staffing because these programs were less structured and depended upon their membership to carry out activities. It appears, however, that volunteer staff were important in all three levels of senior centers.

In terms of scheduling, there was a direct, positive relationship between number of days and hours senior centers were open and level of program. In fact, the mean scores for days and hours open were very close to those proposed in the classification. The only difference was in the number of hours Level Two programs were open (5.5 hours) which exceeded the three (or more) hours suggested in the classification. This finding further lends support to viewing congregate meal sites as more than single purpose programs.

Finally, the results somewhat support the senior center classification in terms of funding sources. In the classification, the funding sources became more diverse as the level of program increased. The results showed that Level Two and Three programs were funded by a variety of sources, primarily federal and local monies. Level One programs overwhelmingly were funded by contributions and/or dues. Interestingly, however, contributions and/or dues also was one of the main sources of revenue for Level Two and Three programs. Perhaps this suggests the willingness and also the necessity of these programs to provide some of their own funding.

There are three implications that can be drawn from this study. First, the "senior center" may be a much broader program than ever realized before. Older people may not make definite distinctions between the traditional senior center, congregate meal programs and senior clubs. They may see *all* of these programs as places to go for a range of services and activities. For example, older people may not distinguish between meals provided by a government-funded congregate meal program and those provided by themselves through senior club potluck dinners. In the study, many respondents listed potluck dinners as an "other" program, while some perhaps mistakenly thought congregate meals and potluck dinners were the same thing. Nevertheless, potluck dinners meet many of the same nutritional and social needs of congregate meals, except the food is provided by the participants themselves. Regardless of *who* provides the service to the elderly, critical needs are being met. Viewing senior centers from this broadened perspective is important in order to have an accurate picture of service providers and recipients within a given area.

A second implication concerns the need for practitioners and policymakers to tap the resources available within senior clubs and organizations. Senior clubs, as well as other senior programs, often have been criticized for their social and "frivolous" nature (Eklund, 1969; London, 1970). However, results from this study indicated that these programs were providing some needed activities and services for their members. For example, over 30 of the Level One programs had outreach and information and referral services. On a returned questionnaire, a senior club leader from a small rural community provided an explanation for this finding:

> Our club has its own form of information and referral service. If a person has a problem, he or she tells someone in our club and all of us do the best we can to solve it. We also have our own transportation service by volunteering to pick up members for meetings as well as for shopping and doctor's appointments.

It is apparent that some senior clubs are providing an informal support system for their members. With current budget cuts, efforts such as these will need to increase. Practitioners and policymakers can assist these efforts by keeping senior club leaders informed about the needs of local elderly and by getting their input into decisions regarding service delivery.

A final implication concerns the need to match level of senior center program to the needs of older people within a respective community or area. The findings showed that programs at all levels were essentially "senior centers." Thus, each community would need to decide on the level of program that would serve as the most effective focal point for service delivery. For example, in some communities, a variety of senior clubs might be sufficient for serving older people. This appears to be the case within some of Iowa's tiny, homogeneous rural communities. In larger, more diverse communities, a network of congregate meal programs and/or multi-purpose senior centers may be needed. While community size may be an important variable in this decision making, characteristics and needs of the older people also would be important factors. This is particularly true concerning communities that have diverse socio-economic and ethnic older populations. On balance, the matching process would allow a "fit" between, on the one hand, the characteristics and needs of the older people, and on the other hand, the level of program provided. More importantly, the matching process might prevent the development of severely underutilized government programs.

In conclusion, this paper has presented a broadened view of senior centers as group-based programs for the elderly. Future research efforts may require a further refinement of the classification of senior center programs, different sampling techniques, and more rigorous statistical treatments.

REFERENCE NOTES

1. The Task Force on Senior Center Development. Senior center programs—an issue paper. Report prepared for Administration on Aging, Department of Health, Education, and Welfare, Washington, DC, 1978.

2. Ralston, P.A. Identification and description of senior center programs in Iowa. Final Report. Iowa Commission on the Aging, Des Moines, Iowa, 1979.

NOTES

3. *Drop-in facilities* - Space available for older persons to socialize or do other activities. (It was felt that drop-in facilities could be considered a service to those who may not want to participate in organized activities within a senior center.) *Recreation/leisure* - Activities for older people designed for relaxation or entertainment purposes. *Information and referral* - Information giving is a service where an older person receives information in response to an expressed need concerning the opportunities and services available. Referral is a service given when an individual's needs are determined through an assessment and the person is directed to a particular resource or choice of resources (Holmes & Holmes, 1979). *Transportation* - Services for older persons who are limited in mobility, lack access to public transportation, or who are unable to pay transportation costs. These services are provided to groups of individuals seeking access to service agencies as well as personal services such as shopping, physician appointments, etc. (Holmes & Holmes, 1979). *Escort* - Services for older persons who require assistance on a one-to-one basis in getting to service agencies or taking care of personal business (e.g., apartment searching, hospital visitations, etc.) because of physical or mental impairment, timidity or fear for personal security, and who may additionally need assistance in presenting their circumstances to agency personnel (Holmes & Holmes, 1979). *Health* - Services provided so that older people can achieve and maintain the highest possible degree of physical and emotional well-being. Specific services include health maintenance (e.g., health screening, physical examinations, immunizations), health education, supervised exercise, and health-related assistance and instructions (e.g., filling out forms for Medicare and Medicaid) (Holmes & Holmes, 1979). *Education* - Activities designed to increase knowledge and skills or to change attitudes of older people. Activities may involve group, one-to-one, or self-directed instruction. *Outreach* - Services where older people, particularly the isolated and impaired, are identified to apprise them of available services and activities. (Holmes & Holmes, 1979). *Congregate meals* - Service where meals are provided for older people in a group setting.

4. Because the 1978 amendments to the Act consolidated nutrition and senior center funding into Title III, respondents associated these funding sources with the old Titles V and VII.

REFERENCES

Administration on Aging. Program development handbook for state and area agencies on multipurpose senior centers. Washington, DC: Department of Health, Education, and Welfare, 1977.

Demko, D. J. Utilization, attrition and the senior center. *Journal of Gerontological Social Work,* 1979, *2,* 87-93.

Downing, J. Factors affecting the selective use of a social club for the aged. *Journal of Gerontology,* 1957, *12,* 81-84.

Eklund, L. Aging and the field of education. In J. W. Riley, Jr. and M. E. Johnson (Eds.), *Aging and Society,* New York: Russell Sage Foundation, 1969.

Frankel, G. The multi-purpose senior citizens center. *Gerontologist,* 1966, *6,* 23-27.

Hanssen, A. M., Meima, N. J., Buckspan, L. M., Henderson, B. E., Helbig, T. L., & Zarit, S. H. Correlates of senior citizen participation. *Gerontologist,* 1978, *18,* 193-199.

Harris, L. & Associates, Inc., *The myth and reality of aging in America.* Washington, DC: National Council on Aging, Inc., 1975.

Holmes, M. B., & Holmes, D. *Handbook of human services for older persons.* New York: Human Sciences Press, 1979.

Hoppa, M. E., & Roberts, G. D. Implications of the activity factor. *Gerontologist,* 1974, *14,* 331-335.

Jones, E. E. An analysis of adult education programs in selected senior citizen centers in Rhode Island (Doctoral dissertation, Columbia University Teachers College, 1976). *Dissertation Abstracts International,* 1976, *37,* 5529-A.

Kutner, B., Fanshel, D., Togo, A. M., & Langner, T. S. *Five hundred over sixty.* New York: Russell Sage, 1956.

London, J. The social setting for adult education. In R. M. Smith, G. F. Aker & J. R. Kidd (Eds.), *Handbook of adult education.* New York: Macmillan Co., 1970.

National Institute of Senior Centers. *Senior center standards, guidelines for practice.* Washington, DC: National Council on the Aging, Inc., 1978.

Pierce, C. H. Recreation for the elderly: Activity participation at a senior citizen center. *Gerontologist,* 1975, *15,* 202-205.

Rosow, I. *Social integration of the aged.* New York: Free Press, 1967.

Taietz, P. Two conceptual models of the senior center. *Journal of Gerontology,* 1976, *31,* 219-222.

Tissue, T. Social class and the senior citizen center. *Gerontologist,* 1971, *11,* 196-200.

Intergenerational Programming: An Adopt-a-Grandparent Program in a Retirement Community

Ruth E. Dunkle
Betsey G. Mikelthun

Numerous studies over the last 25 years have explored the attitudes of the young to the old (Axelrod and Eisdorfer, 1961; Frake, 1957; Golde and Kogan, 1959; Kogan and Shelton, 1962; Tuckman and Lorge, 1958; Ivester and King, 1977; Thomas and Yamamoto, 1975; Hickey and Kalish, 1968). More recently some limited attention has been directed toward determining the attitudes of the elderly toward the young (Cryns and Monk, 1972; Seefeldt, Jantz, Galper and Serock, 1977; Seefeldt, Jantz, Serock and Bredekamp, 1980). These studies highlight existing stereotypes and the concomitant problems. Neugarten, for example, found that

> stereotypes about aging and the aged create a particularly complex set of problems. In addition to making us fear aging, the stereotypes lead to a decisiveness in society at large that has been called ageism that is negative or hostile attitudes between age groups that lead to socially destructive competition. (1976)

One potential result is an isolated older population that is rejected by younger age groups. This particular suggestion implies that the elderly are not isolated by choice and would interact with younger people if the opportunity were available. This view, however, has not been supported by other research. Seefeldt, Jantz, Serock and

Ruth E. Dunkle, PhD and Betsey G. Mikelthun, MSSA are with the School of Applied Social Sciences, Case Western Reserve University, Cleveland, Ohio 44106.

Bredekamp (1980) found that the elderly's attitudes towards the young are not always positive.

The attitude of the elderly towards the young is a result of their view of themselves (Bennet and Eckman, 1973). Hickey and Kalish (1968) state that the adult population including the elderly themselves see old people as living in a social climate which is not conducive to feelings of usefulness, adequacy, and security.

The present study focuses on the effect of the Adopt-A-Grandparent/Grandchild Program on the retirement community, the school children, and the parents and/or families of the children who participate. Although foster grandparent programs have developed in response to the need for intergenerational programming, none have examined the reasons why some older adults choose to participate while others do not.

Interviews were conducted with a random sample of nonparticipating residents in the retirement community to assess their attitudes toward the program and why they hadn't participated. Former participants were interviewed regarding their feelings toward the program and their reasons for ceasing to participate. Observation, questionnaires, and diaries kept by older participants were used to evaluate the effect on the adults involved in the program.

Participant observation, taped interviews, and diaries kept by the grandchildren provided data on the children's experiences in the program. In addition, at the end of each school year, the children who had participated were tested regarding their attitude toward the elderly, as was a control group from the same grade but a different classroom. Parents of the children participating in the program also were asked to fill out questionnaires at the end of the school year.

The objectives of the Adopt-A-Grandparent/Grandchild Program were as follows:

1. To provide elderly persons in an age segregated environment the opportunity for a long term intergenerational experience;
2. To allow children an experience of sharing a relationship with an older person and to enhance their perception of aging;
3. To explore why the elderly participate in such a program.

This paper will review the development of the program as well as describe issues of participation of old and the young and issues of intergenerational programming.

Program Setting and Participants

The retirement community that sponsored the program is a non-profit multilevel care facility located in Cleveland, Ohio. Participants were recruited from the independent living unit which has 154 housing units as well as from the Day Enrichment Center, a day care program for mild to moderately impaired elders residing in the community.

Residents of the retirement community and the Day Enrichment Program were invited to join the program by an announcement in the weekly calendar of events. If interested, they were to sign up on a centrally located bulletin board. Very few showed initial interest. Further recruitment by the Director of Activities identified fourteen participants. The initial reluctance to join the program may have been due to the impersonal contact through the calendar of events. Only with the personal encouragement of the Activities Director did people join.

The initial reluctance to participate in the program was an unexpected response. Although residents are typically informed of programs through the bulletin board, the nature of the adopted grandparent program seemed to elicit more reluctance and/or ambivalence than the staff of the retirement community had seen previously. This program was the first one involving children that required a commitment from the older resident to participate. Other programs involving children usually only required the resident to be a passive audience, as with Christmas Sing, etc. Possibly, the residents felt more vulnerable due to the uncertainty of program expectations, i.e., time commitment, expectations of the child, and the nature of activities in which they would be expected to engage.

The three-year program began in 1977 with 14 second graders from a local elementary school. Students participated on a voluntary basis with the approval of their parents. The number of participants was limited to 14 during the first year and 13 in subsequent years due to transportation restrictions. Table 1 identifies the number of persons involved in the program over a three-year period.

For the first two years, a second grade class was involved, but during the third year of the program, a group of fourth graders was involved because the teacher responsible for the program was moved from second grade to the fourth grade. There were also more "grandparents" than "grandchildren" involved, to offset absences due to poor health.

TABLE 1

Involvement for Three Years

Year	Grade	Number of Children	New Children	Number of Adults	New Adults
1977–1978	2nd	14	14	18*	18
1978–1979	2nd	13	12	16*	10
1979–1980	4th	13	8	15	2
	Total	40	34	49	30

*There were 4 adult substitutes in 1977–
1978 and 2 adult substitutes in 1978–1979.

During the course of the three years of the program 30 different elderly persons were involved directly with the children. Twenty five were female, five were male. Two of the women participants had never married. Four of the participants, two women and two men, though having been married, had no children. The remaining twenty-four were married and had both children and grandchildren. Three participants died in the course of the program's first three years.

It is interesting to note the consistency of grandparents during the program years. There appears to have been a commitment to the program by these residents even when they could not be committed to the same child each year. Ten of the 18 old people who started in the program in 1977 continued the following year; in 1979, 13 of the 15 residents continued in the program.

Drop-Out Rate

One interesting dimension of the program was that "grand-parents" had the opportunity of continuing for the three-year period, while this was not the case for the children during the first two years. Those "grandparents" not continuing in the program were interviewed. Thirteen elders chose to limit their involvement in the program. Six dropped out of the program for health reasons. Of the four who participated for two of the three years, three stopped for health reasons and two ultimately returned when their health improved. The fourth person dropped out of the program the second year because of other responsibilities but did return to the program for the third year. The remainder of the people who dropped out of the program did so for a variety of reasons. In the third year, however, eight of the fourth grade students who had participated during the first year as second graders chose to participate again. Two people dropped the program after one year because the day was changed and they were busy on the new day. One woman realized that she didn't feel comfortable with children any more. One man felt that the situation was too contrived and didn't allow for real closeness. One woman felt that the relationships were too superficial and that there wasn't enough depth. Another woman felt that there was too much depth and that she was getting too involved with the child and his family.

Program Activities

During the first year of the program, the children were encouraged to bring items that they treasured to share with their grandparents. The children brought their favorite books and games and told their grandparents about them. On a few occasions activities were planned by the activities director for grandparents and grandchildren as a group instead of the typical one-to-one arrangement. These included exercise day, a Christmas party, bingo, a Valentine's party, crafts day, a continental breakfast and magic show that included the children's parents, and an end of the year potluck picnic.

CHILDREN'S ATTITUDES TOWARD THE ELDERLY

An effort was made to measure the children's attitude toward the elderly during the first two program years. The second grade children participating in the program and two control groups from other second grade classes in the same school were orally administered a true/false attitude test. Compared with those in the control groups, fewer participants in the program appear to have stereotypes. A more difficult true/false test was administered to the fourth grades (Table 3). Results for these groups of fourth graders are similar to those of the second graders. Those children who chose to participate in the program seem to have fewer misconceptions about older people. The fourth grade program participants, however, seemed to be more dramatically affected than were the second grade participants. This may show an increased stereotypic reaction to older persons with age. Thus, the older children exposed to older persons show a marked reduction in their misconceptions of the aged.

The impact of self-selection of the students participating in the program should be addressed. The children involved in the program may have joined because they held fewer stereotypic impressions of what older people were like, but it should be noted that the control

TABLE 2

Second Grade True/False Test*

		Participants True False ($\underline{N}$ = 24)		Nonparticipants True False ($\underline{N}$ = 24)	
1.	You can learn from older people.	24	0	21	3
2.	Older people never have any fun.	0	24	3	21
3.	Older people are boring and uninteresting.	0	24	3	21
4.	Older people have had wrinkles all their lives.	1	23	5	19
5.	Older people are unattractive.	1	23	4	20
6.	Older people need exercise.	24	0	20	4
7.	You should leave older people alone because they like being by themselves.	0	24	7	17

*Two second grade groups are combined, as are the control groups.

TABLE 3

Fourth Grade True/False Test

	Participants True False ($\underline{N}$ = 12)		Nonparticipants True False ($\underline{N}$ = 12)	
	True	False	True	False
1. In older people, the senses of touch, pain taste, and smell are all reduced.	4	8	8	4
2. Older people are unattractive.	0	12	4	8
3. An older person is beyond the age when he/she can contribute to society.	1	11	5	7
4. Achievement and being successful are not important to older people.	0	12	5	7
5. As people age, they tend to become more demanding, complaining, irritable, fault-finding, and suspicious.	0	12	7	5
6. All people when they get old, become senile.	1	11	5	7
7. Different parts of the body age at different rates.	8	4	12	0
8. Older people are more vulnerable to diseases and accidents.	7	5	10	2

group was drawn from another classroom and most likely included children with a broad range of beliefs about the elderly.

Older Persons Viewed as Different

When the children were asked how older people were different from them, there seemed to be a difference in responses given by second and fourth graders. Second graders typically made general observations about the physical attributes of old age, e.g., "older people have gray hair and wrinkly skin"; "they carry canes and can't walk as fast"; "sometimes they can't see or hear as well as we can"; and "they have big veins in their hands." The fourth graders responded in terms of experiential differences. One student pointed to the fact that older people don't go to school as she does and that older people talk about the past a lot. Another child mentioned that "they seem to be more gentle," and a third said that "some are funnier."

How are older people similar? "They're people too"; "They can do anything you can do"; "they're the same, but a different person." These answers again point to the commonality discovered by these fourth grade youngsters. Other similarities were that older people have the same interests, act like friends, and that both age groups can learn things.

What will you be like when you are older? Several second and fourth graders said the obvious, that someday they would be older themselves. Some indicated that they thought they would be similar in some way or other to the adopted grandparent they had had. One girl said she thought she would be "grumpy." When asked why she thought that, she replied, "Because when you're young and grumpy, when you get older you'll be grumpy."

Parents

Each year the parents were asked to fill out an evaluation, and 35 to 40 possible questionnaires were filled out and returned in the three years of the program. Parents were asked to evaluate what they felt their child had learned from this experience. Several mentioned that their children had learned they could have fun with older people. Parents also noted that they had learned to share not only tangible items but also love and time. Some children learned concrete things, e.g., older people are interested in children, and older people often have fewer activities. Others learned that everyone must slow down as they get older. One parent said that her child learned he will not be young forever. Another parent said, "she learned that being old is not dead. People continue to have dreams, hopes and desires to do things as usual."

REASONS FOR OLD PERSONS' INVOLVEMENT

One aspect of this project was to determine why certain older persons choose to participate in the program and others did not. A random sample of nonparticipating older persons (16% of N = 31) eligible to participate at the beginning of third year in the retirement community were interviewed concerning their lack of involvement. Of the 31 persons interviewed, 29 were female, 25 were married and 22 had children and grandchildren. Ages ranged from 65 to 96. Even though these people did not choose to participate in the program, several did feel that they would in the future (16.1%). Another 19.3% thought that they might join in the future, whereas 6.4% said that, even though they did not want to be a grandparent, they would be interested in being involved in a peripheral way, e.g., attending the parties (Table 4). Further, these nonparticipants were asked about benefits of participating. Many could see benefits of the program and responded with more than one answer (Table 5).

In stating the positive aspects of the program, grandparents identified slightly more with the children than for themselves. Perhaps it is easier to see the benefits of something to someone other than oneself. Several spoke of the opportunity to be with children as good, invigorating, or giving them a new zest for living. Many spoke of the relationships as being good for both the children and the grand-

TABLE 4

Reasons for Nonparticipation

($\underline{N}$ = 31)

1. 32.2% -- were too busy, had no time to participate.

2. 29.0% -- activities did not appeal to them.

3. 25.8% -- cited health reasons.

4. 16.1% -- were not interested in being involved.

5. 12.9% -- did not feel comfortable with children.

6.   9.6% -- mentioned involvement with their own families.

7.   6.4% -- did not comprehand the question (had orientation problems).

8.   3.2% -- did not know anything about the program and had not
             participated for that reason.

Due to multiple responses total is
more than 100%

TABLE 5

Benefits of Participating As
Suggested by Nonparticipants

Response	N
1. Contact with younger generation.	12
2. Something to look forward to.	8
3. Good if no grandchildren of your own.	5
4. Feelings of usefulness or being important.	5
5. Being involved with others besides self.	4
6. Cure for loneliness.	3
7. Enjoyment.	2
8. Exposure to other racial groups.	1
Total	40

parents, and of the benefits of exposing two generations to each other. Benefits to the children that were cited included awakening their concern for older people and promoting positive feelings toward older people as well as teaching them to respect older people. One of the more complex responses on the positive aspects was, "It is a very helpful program to our age group. I think we naturally are inclined to shut ourselves in with a feeling of, 'well, it's all over.' It brings back your own childhood with memories of positive, negative, humorous experiences and comparing them with the reactions of the 'new age' child. There really is not too great a difference. It makes it possible to reach out to your child in spite of age differences." Another woman indicated a positive aspect of the program as simply "affection directed to this grandma." Four people spoke of the interracial benefits. "I think it helped black and white to realize we are all the same, you never think of color."

When asked what the negative aspects of the program were the majority of grandparents answered, "none." Several replied, "The time was too short." Other comments included, "I wish more Judson Park residents could participate," and "I am sure there is always room for improvement in anything; however, I was never a group worker and would not know the negatives."

Participants in the program tended to see benefits primarily to the children. Nonparticipants spoke of benefits to the participants. The self-selection of grandparents may explain this difference. Possibly, the older participants joined due to their interest in children. On the other hand the nonparticipants focused on themselves and, therefore, were less inclined to engage in a program designed around the interest of the children.

ISSUES FOR INTERGENERATIONAL PROGRAMMING

The major contribution of this study for future program development are in two areas: recruitment and participation.

Recruitment

The initial reluctance to sign up for this program can be explained from the findings of a study by Irving Rosow (1967). He found that relations to children by older persons are fraught with anxiety, distortion and denial, as older persons make an effort to reassure themselves. Furthermore, the study by Seefeldt et al. (1980) pointed to certain factors among older persons that are related to positive attitudes toward children and that mitigate negative feelings, namely, degree of knowledge, education and contact with children; as the "grandparents" related to their grandchildren, their fears receded, resulting in their beliefs that the children really benefited from the program. On the other hand, the nonparticipants continued to focus on the older person's benefit from participation, possibly a reflection on their continued anxiety.

These views on recruitment suggest that a more active face-to-face recruitment is necessary in programs involving ongoing contact with children. Other techniques to reduce anxiety also should be employed. Educating the potential older participants as to specific activities of program and time will help. Possibly, a planning meeting could be held to inform potential participants, thus reducing the threat of commitment to the program and ultimately a child.

Participation

When the nonparticipants were asked why they did not participate the most frequent reason was lack of time. Possibly, these people are already active and do not feel the need to join another activity. On the other hand, 29% said that the activities of the program did not appeal to them. Choosing activities that are of greater interest would be helpful. Once again, a planning meeting of potential participants would aid in the identification of meaningful programs. The age of the children also may be relevant. Whereas 46% of the nonparticipants identified second and fourth graders as the children best suited to participate in such a program, 14% felt that the children should be younger; 35% wanted them to be older. These differences indicate that older persons have a variety of interests and that future programs should include a wider age range of children.

CONCLUSION

Providing relevant programs to the elderly is a needed service. Understanding why certain older persons choose to participate and why others do not provides clues to meet this goal. The findings of the intergenerational programming of an adopted grandparent program indicate that this type of program can be meaningful to certain types of older persons and children.

REFERENCES

Axelrod, S., and Eisdorfer, C. Attitudes toward older people: An empirical analysis of the stimulus group validity of the Tuckman-Large questionnaire. *Journal of Gerontology,* 1961, *16,* 75-80.

Bennet, R., and Eckman, J. Attitudes toward aging: A critical examination of recent literature and implications for future research, in C. Eisdorfer and M. P. Lawton (eds.), *The psychology of adult development and aging.* Washington: American Psychological Association, 1973.

Cryns, A., and Monk, A. Attitudes of the aged toward the young: A multivariate study in intergenerational perception. *Journal of Gerontology,* 1972, *27,* 107-112.

Drake, J. T. Some factors influencing student attitudes toward older people. *Social Forces,* 1957, *35,* 266-271.

Golde, P., and Kogan, W. A sentence completion procedure for assessing attitudes toward old people. *Journal of Gerontology,* 1959, *14,* 355-363.

Hickey, T., & Kalish, R. Young people's perceptions of adults. *Journal of Gerontology,* 1968, 215-219.

Ivester, C., and King, K. Attitudes of adolescents toward the aged. *The Gerontologist,* 1977, *1,* 85-89.

Kogan, N., and Shelton, F. C. Beliefs about "old people;" A comparative study of older and younger samples. *Journal of Genetic Psychology,* 1962, *100,* 93-111.

Neugarten, B. L. Grow old along with me! The best is yet to be. In S. White (ed.), *Human development in today's world.* Boston: Little, Brown, 1976.

Rosow, I. *Social integration of the aged.* New York: The Free Press, 1967.

Seefeldt, C., Jantz, R., Galper, A., and Serock, K. Using pictures to explore children's attitudes toward the elderly. *The Gerontologist,* 1977, *17,* 506-512.

Seefeldt, C., Jantz, R., Serock, K., and Bredekamp, S. Elderly persons' attitudes toward children. Findings from research project funded by the American Association Retired Persons, National Retired Teachers Association, Andrus Foundation, 1980.

Thomas, E., and Yamamoto, K. Attitudes toward age: An exploration in school age children. *International Journal of Aging and Human Development,* 1975, *6,* 117-129.

Tuckman, J., and Lorge, I. Attitudes toward aging of individuals with experiences with the aged. *Journal of Genetic Psychology,* 1958, *92,* 199-205.

Recreational Travel
with the Elderly:
Some Observations

Ursula A. Falk

It is my privilege to take at least one two-week tour annually with a group of elderly persons. During the past eight years I have escorted a total of 715 older individuals on fifteen different vacations averaging from five to fifteen days in duration. These folks ranged from sixty-five to ninety-five and are in various states of health. The majority view their compatriots as old—"that old man," "that senile old woman," but exclude themselves from that category, saying, "I would like it here if there weren't so many old people around."

This year, as last, we chose a Miami Beach resort hotel which is very accommodating to our many and varied needs. The group of fifteen travelers were mainly people of moderate means although one woman in the group is wealthy. All of them are extremely frugal, afraid that they will outlast their money, whether this be real or imaginary. They are simultaneously parenting and have the desire to be parented. Such comments as: "The other hotel is better since the owners are like a papa and a mama" typify this. They usually "hang on" to the escort, demand much of the waiters, maids and other hotel personnel and when ignored, pressure the travel escort to meet their demands for them. They run to their escort with every bruise and ache, asking for protection and care. They feel that they must eat as much as their stomach can hold in order to "get their money's worth." When served family style each will heap his plate until there is nothing left for those at the other end of the table.

Ursula A. Falk, MSW, EdD is a certified social worker and lecturer in Gerontology Sociology Dept. at the State University College and Canisius College; and nursing home consultant at Newfane Health Facility, Niagara Geriatric Center, and Presbyterian Homes, in Buffalo, N.Y.

Preoccupation with the gastro-intestinal tract is always present. "My bowels haven't moved in four days." Three or more helpings of prunes plus tablespoons of Metamucil are not unusual as a small part of the breakfast fare of one of my followers. That, preceded and followed by hot and cold cereal, smoked salmon, two or more rolls, cream cheese, eggs, juice, "and a couple or so small pieces of cake," with many cups of coffee, call a great deal of attention to the intestines and adjoining organs. Seeing something ordered by another customer makes the onlooker immediately compete for that extra helping of food. Minimizing the intake, as the person later describes his meal, are all a part of the fun! A number of would-be heart attacks have been known to occur after one or another such meal.

Most of the people in the group are always very flattering to me and "honey-bunch," "sweetheart," and "darling" are frequently used terms. If they praise me a great deal they believe that they have bought insurance and will be well cared for and spared from all misfortune. They also freely pepper their conversations with G'd willing, G'd forbid and "we should only stay well to be able to come next time."

A great deal of unburdening occurs between the traveler and the escort. The senior feels free to share intimate details of her life. The children that are always spoken of as "angels" and "dolls" become real human beings who are sometimes neglectful and uncaring. The fact that there is a physical distance between their child and their vacation spot facilitates an open expression of feelings.

There is a great need to be touched and to touch. The need for human contact and warmth is very noticeable. Added to this is the physical pulling and "grabbing at" the escort. By feeling a younger stronger arm they seem to feel a bit more alive themselves. They do not have the opportunity afforded the younger person for physical contact with other human beings.

Sex is decidedly a part of the seniors' life at any age. Singles will try hard to attract each other. Single women will attempt to gain the attention of the few men at the hotel and the men will try to attract younger women. A seventy-year-old gentleman proposed marriage to me two days after our Miami arrival. He approached me because, "I don't like old ladies, and you're still young." When younger persons refuse to become amorously involved with the elderly men they will turn to the younger-looking of their peers. The "young-old" like to dance. Since there are so many more females than males, the men often have many dancing partners in the course of one evening. Those women who are not asked to dance by the opposite sex will dance with one another, thus having some fairly close physical contact with another person. The few intact older couples that were on my latest trip enjoy "normal" sexuality. My room was adjoining that of a married pair. The man is ninety-two and the woman eighty-five. He is very much physically debilitated and walks very slowly with a cane. In fact, he needed a wheel chair at the airport since he cannot ambulate over longer distances. He is extremely hard of hearing, thus his requests were clearly heard by me. He had intercourse twice during the first ten days of vacation. One night his wife loudly refused him—"please, no, I'm tired." This rejection was repeated at least four times that night since the man was very persistent and obviously made his last attempt at 3:00 A.M. Another couple on this last trip were celebrating their forty-fifth wedding anniversary and told me they were planning to "have a good time" just like on their honeymoon. Other trips found some single folk taking single rooms and inviting "boy" or "girl" friends in for a night.

There is a feeling of security for the elderly in traveling in a group with people that they have known for a time. Since hotel management and other travel personnel are much more able to ignore the individual elderly traveler, he or she feels much better taken care of in a group where a known escort is available to meet the various individual needs. Multitudinous requests will be made of the escort and promises of future trips will be made to her: "everyone will go with you next time." This was frequently uttered and was generally followed or preceded by a request. There is the constant "do for me" appeal and the same folks praise the escort incessantly. The most frequent praises are pronounced by the person who is generally rejected by his peers. A deaf woman, for example, who was ignored not only by her roommate, but by other members of the group, lauded my efforts without cessation (a request for help and attention on her part—"if I praise you enough you won't disappoint me and be my friend and mentor"). I played Scrabble with this woman and lost to her. This afforded her status and attention which she obviously needed.

Assurances that a bargain was had, was another phenomenon. Repeated requests for comparative shopping for other hotels was a part of this venture. Only when they were shown on paper that ours was the most reasonably priced hotel did the travelers appear somewhat satisfied. "Try this other hotel around the corner—it might be cheaper."

The majority of the elderly which I have accompanied have difficulty tipping their hotel servants. The gratuities are almost non-existent. They want to be assured that they do not need to leave anything for the personnel and use the escort to stamp approval for their inability to part with their funds. The group generally does leave the waiter and bus boy about ten cents per day per person and expects much service and gratitude for this. I have learned to caution the group not to leave their combined tip until the last meal, otherwise the service becomes extremely poor. There is much competition as to who will present the waiter with the group tip and who will collect it from the fellow travelers. Peg, one of our group members, insisted that she had asked people for the tips before Ellen did and now the latter "is bossing things." Again, this is a status problem, each wanting to be important and the supervisor over the money.

In the resort hotels which cater mainly to the elderly (young people are seldom seen in these, since they do not care to associate with the elderly) there are a number of confused people. One man, for example, who came with a group, left and was not seen again until he was picked up days later by a kindly traveler, miles from the hotel. One man approached everyone with "woo, woo" and then made nonsense rhymes into the faces of other vacationers. Another very grotesque looking lady dragged her cursing ninety year old lame husband on the dance floor. Others tell almost their entire life story to all willing or unwilling listeners. Still others will give bizarre performances on stage during "showtime."

A social hostess is provided by all hotels which we frequented in our travels. She is usually a saccharine sweet middle aged woman who can become very curt at a moment's notice. A number of the elderly do not openly object to this behavior and accept it most of the time. The social hostess, on the other hand, is plagued by unrealistic demands and is criticized by the movies she brings or the third rate entertainers which are affordable.

Trips mean a great deal to many elderly folk. It gives them something positive to look toward, something to plan for in the future and something to talk about when it is over. It gives them an opportunity to be away from their often drab environment and affords them a fresh outlook. I have found traveling with the elderly an interesting and unique experience.

ADDITIONAL RESOURCES FOR WORKING WITH THE "WELL ELDERLY"

AGING PARENTS. Pauline K. Ragan (Ed.). *University of Southern California Press, 1979. 295 pages. (Paperback, with no price indicated).*

This book is a collection of reports, statistics and research in the field of gerontology. Most of the chapters were developed from presentations at the "You and Your Aging Parents" Conference at the Andrus Gerontology Center in May, 1978.

The chapters present various aspects of the aging process, debunk myths of aging and provide solid research information in the field of gerontology.

In the preface, editor Pauline Ragan states: "The collection has been designed for use by individuals with personal interests, by professionals involved in counseling and research, and as a textbook for classes and workshops."

Several chapters are scholarly and statistical, not meant for the lay person; but the majority of the articles, written by experts, present current and viable alternatives for those people who work, live or care for the elderly.

Particularly noteworthy are the myths of aging that are dispelled by several authors. Most of the experts did find that the majority of adult children are actively involved in caring for their elderly parents. Three-quarters of those elderly with children see them almost daily or at least weekly.

The fallacy of role reversal, where parent and adult child exchange roles, is put to rest. Instead, several authors discuss the aspect of filial maturity whereby the parent and adult child assume interdependent roles.

Several experts encourage gerontological professionals to con-

111

sider the entire family unit whenever counseling is involved. The life of each family member impinges upon every other life in that family. All too often professionals have dealt only with the problems of the older parent and have not considered the desires of other family members.

Professionals will find this book an informative handbook of current research. In addition, it is a book that can help those adult children who are working through their own crises with aging parents.

Sue Ann Luxa, MA
Littleton, Colorado

AN EASIER WAY: HANDBOOK FOR THE ELDERLY & HANDICAPPED. Jean Vieth Sargent. *Walker & Company, 1982. 218 pages. $12.95.*

> . . . an eminently useful book. Literally scores of ideas, some of them quite ingenious, have been gathered, offering disabled or frail individuals means of independently performing otherwise hard-to-do tasks. . .this is an easy to use handbook and highly recommended.
>
> —*Library Journal*

Anyone concerned with the care of the elderly or handicapped will find this collection of over 200 gadgets, hints, suggestions and information an invaluable find. Simple devices, many of which can be ordered by mail or made easily at home, are designed to facilitate those everyday tasks most of us take for granted, but which present problems for the disabled. Tap turners, an apron for the one-handed that does not need tying on, color coded clothing tags in Braille to help the fashion-conscious blind, writing aids for arthritic hands—these devices and others can lead the way to greater independence and self-reliance for the infirm.

The book is divided into subject areas (Cooking and Cleaning; Dressing and Grooming; Keeping Warm; Moving About; Visual Aids; Wheelchair Specials, etc.), with large, clear type and helpful diagrammatic pictures. Devices are keyed to mail-order resources and supplemented by a list of organizations and publications, all designed to increase the elderly or handicapped person's flexibility and comfort.

Jean Vieth Sargent writes a column in two Iowa newspapers (Cedar Rapids and Ames) under the same title, "An Easier Way," and the suggestions in this helpful book are the cream of her collection.

An Occupational Therapist at the Northeast Home Health Care, Fort Collins, CO, offered these additional words regarding this book.

> I passed the book around amongst the staff here and we're ordering one for our patients to check out. I was a bit sceptical of a "How To" book for the handicapped, because individual abilities and involvements can vary so much from person to person, even with the same diagnosis. However, this book really approaches, by way of its style, adaptations very well. Certainly, organization by subject rather than by diagnosis helps this to happen. The large print and the simplicity of "tips" are excellent! Thanks for sharing it with me!

COUNSELING ELDERS AND THEIR FAMILIES. John Herr and John Weakland. *Springer Publishing Company. 1979. $16.50. Hardback.*

It has, in the past, been difficult to find books that are relevant and helpful in the field of counseling the elderly and aging. This is a fairly new area of study in looking at the human condition. This book is well written and very readable; an excellent guide for persons providing services to the elderly.

The first section deals primarily with workers and elderly who seemingly get together in a very haphazard fashion. The professional counselor, or other helper, looks at the elderly and the life traumas and difficulties that the aged/aging face and that must be resolved in counseling. The situation must not deteriorate so that a painful situation becomes worse.

This section of the book discusses how to start a counseling ses-

sion, from the physical set-up to the process used in the beginning
meeting. A most important point that is here made, is what NOT to
do.

Part two of the book gives the background on the theory and practice of family therapy and includes many helpful excerpts from research done in this area. Included also are many demonstrations of
how family systems theory can be used in working with the elderly.
The interaction between elderly and their families gives many clues
to problems other than those identified by the client.

Part three of this book is an extensive recounting of case studies
that should be most helpful. The focus of the counseling is on the
daily living of the elderly and how to make this point in life worth-
while.

Belle Miran
Geriatric Counselor
Denver, Colorado

THE OLDER ADULT: A PROCESS FOR WELLNESS. Elizabeth
Jane Forbes and Virginia Macken Fitzsimons. *The C. V. Mosby
Company, 1981, 333 pages, $11.95, softcover.*

The Older Adult: A Process for Wellness is an attractively pack-
aged softcovered book that deals with a little of everything concerning the older adult. As its title suggests, the focus is on wellness
rather than a medical or illness model, with goals of prevention,
health maintenance, and maintenance of independence to a max-
imum potential in daily living activities. The book incorporates
some of the most current theories and research as well as provides
much practical information on how to work with the older adult.

The four units of the book are divided up according to the components of the nursing process: Data Collection, Care Planning, Intervention and Evaluation.

The first unit on data collection begins with background to the
nursing process and lists the sources of data as the knowledge base,
nursing history, nursing assessment and nursing diagnosis. The
various theories on aging are introduced: the biologic, the psychological, and the sociological, with the major theories and theorists in

each category. Then, an overview of the anatomy and physiology of the different body systems is presented along with the effects of aging on each system. Pictures, charts and tables lend clarity to this section.

A variety of topics is included in the section on models of care. Several models of nursing care are described, and the use of theory in nursing is explained. A brief review of some of the theories in nursing is presented including Roy's adaptation theory, Roger's holistic model and Gunter's gerontics. Other topics covered in this section are lifestyle models for older adults, cultural influences on family life, and selected living arrangements for older adults.

The levels of health maintenance and how they relate to the older adult are then described. The nursing record, its component parts, among them the nursing history, review of systems, and a detailed health examination which describes normal and abnormal findings is presented. An interesting reading on the historical perspective of physical assessment skills in nursing follows which shows that rather than being a new, innovative role for nursing, historically it has been within the framework of nursing.

Nursing diagnosis is discussed as the last step of data collection. An explanation of nursing diagnosis, levels, clinical application and use as a standard of care as developed by the American Nurses' Association is included. A clear and complete sample case study with an operational description of the nursing process through the first and second ANA Standards of Gerontological Nursing Practice is provided. Then two selected readings on "Classifying Nursing Diagnoses" and "Why Nursing Diagnosis?" are helpful in covering the issue.

The unit on care planning starts with the role of self-esteem and nursing. The importance of job satisfaction with burnout being on the opposite side of the spectrum is discussed. Then a section on ethics is provided. The International Council of Nurses Code for Nurses, the American Nurses' Association Code of Ethics for Nurses, A Patient's Bill of Rights and Nurses' rights are presented. Exercises in ethical considerations follow for the reader to think about. Caring and assertiveness in nursing are discussed with a description of assertiveness communication techniques. The authors approach assertiveness as an ethical responsibility of nursing which is a new, interesting point of view.

Client care plans are then dealt with; background is provided, advantages discussed and then the importance of their usage in terms of documentation of care is covered. There is an excellent presentation of goals and objectives complete with examples and guidelines. The section then leads into client care conferences; their format and organization, and then to discharge planning as the ultimate goal of client care. Discharge planning is covered by a variety of aspects relating to it.

The next unit on intervention is divided into three parts. The first section is on establishing a relationship through communication; communication theory and process is discussed with a substantial presentation on reality orientation. The last two sections are on modifying nursing approaches for the older adult: the physiological needs and psychosocial needs. The physiological needs of this age group are described with specific, very basic common sense type of interventions designed to meet these needs. The areas range from cosmetics and hair grooming to bowel and bladder, nutrition, housing-shelter, exercise, etc. Selected readings on exercise and sexuality and the aged follow. The psychosocial needs described follow Maslow's hierarchy of needs. Topics here include practicalities on home safety, love and belonging, loneliness, isolation, self-esteem and self-actualization. Community resources to help meet the psychosocial needs are listed. The section is completed with a reading on the morbidity patterns among recently relocated elderly.

The last unit on evaluation deals with the three levels of evaluation. Level I is evaluation as the last step in the nursing process. Level II is the nursing audit. Level III is the utilization review plan. The who, what, when, where, why and how of each of the levels are discussed with forms and worksheets included.

The three appendices are "On being a good listener," a brief explanation of Medicare and a directory of state agencies on aging and regional offices.

The book is not meant as a textbook in gerontological nursing, but rather as a resource to those students involved in studying care of the older adult as well as the nurse in clinical practice who is caring for the older adult. It is also recommended for those nurses interested in continuing education. The book serves these purposes. The topics covered in the book are varied; most of them are not in depth. At the end of each chapter there is an extensive bibliography for any reader interested in supplementing his knowledge on any of the subjects covered. The book is a valuable resource in familiarizing the reader within the realm of caring for the older adult, and in particular, the well older adult.

Lenore B. Weinstein

THE WIDOW. Mary Clare Powell. *1981. 73 pages. $7.00 plus $1.00 postage for each copy. Softback.*

Having been a widow for ten years, I perhaps had more than a passing interest in this book.

Ms. Powell has put into words, very easily understood, many of the experiences we have all had. She speaks of the first month as being a "numb" time when there is a lot of support, many things to do, and she really didn't lean on people, maybe as much as she could or perhaps should have.

Then follows the fact that "couple friends" sort of disappear. I often wonder why but know this to be a fact.

Volunteer work at a local school and getting close to many children with their problems, soon filled her time. She did not wish to be a burden to her own children, but was there to help them if needed. Eventually she learned to enjoy the freedom of her solitude, doing things when and as she wished. That came with time.

Such things as Senior organizations and retiring to Florida seem to have a place, yet she does not want a whole life of that.

She presents her ideas on such topics as marriage, companionship, and many others. In short, this is a very readable, entertaining book full of one woman's ideas and the way to meet that stage of life we all know as "widowhood." It does not have to be all bad. This book is full of lovely and revealing pictures and excellent reading for anyone, but perhaps more especially, those recently widowed. I recommend it highly!

Hazel F. Kempkes

Bibliography on Activities, Adaptations & Aging of the "Well Elderly"

Aging from Birth to Death, Volume 2: Sociotemporal Perspectives. Edited by Matilda White Riley, Ronald P. Abeles, & Michael S. Teitelbaum. 1982. Westview Press. 228 pages. Hardback. $20.00.

Aging: The Process & the People. Edited by Gene Usdin, MD & Charles J. Hofling, MD. The American College of Psychiatrists. Brunner/Mazel, Publishers. 1978. 248 pages. Hardback. $15.00.

Alternatives to Institutional Care for Older Americans: Practice & Planning. A Conference Report. L.O.C. #72-93731. 1973. Center for the Study of Aging and Human Development, Duke University, Durham, NC 27710. Write for more information.

Becoming Old: An Introduction to Social Gerontology. John C. Morgan. 1979. Springer Publishing Co., NY, NY. Softback. 94 pages. $6.50.

Do it Yourself Again: Self Help Devices for The Stroke Patient. American Heart Association, 44 East 23rd St., NY, NY 10010. Write for more information.

Exercises for the Elderly. Robert H. Jamieson. Emerson Books, Inc. 1982. 158 pages. Hardback. Large print. $11.95.

Home Care for The Elderly. Julie Trocchio. CBI Publishing Co., Boston, MA, 161 pages. Softback. $8.95.

Late Adulthood: Perspectives on Human Development. Richard A. Kalish. 1975. Brooks/Cole Publishing Co., Monterey, CA. 133 pages. Softback. $3.95.

Maggie Kuhn on Aging. A dialogue edited by Dieter Hessel. The Westminster Press, Philadelphia. 1977. 140 pages. Softback. $3.95.

Older Persons: Unused Resources for Unmet Needs. Edited by Frank Riessman. 1977. SAGE Publications, Inc., 275 So. Beverly Drive, Beverly Hills, CA 90212. Write for information & further titles.

The One-Hander's Book: A Guide to Activities of Daily Living. Veronica Washam. The John Day Co./An Intext Publisher, NY. 1973. Hardback. $10.00. 126 pages.

The Other Generation Gap: The Middle-Aged & Their Aging Parents. Dr. Stephen Z. Cohen & Bruce Michael Gans. Follett Publishing Co., Chicago. $10.95. Hardback. 290 pages.

Over 50 - So What! Hildegarde. Devin-Adair Co., Old Greenwich, CT. 1963. Hardcover. $5.50. 184 pages.

The First Year: A Retirement Journal. Pearl A. Nelson. Potentials Development for Health & Aging Services, Inc., 775 Main St., Buffalo, NY 14203. 1981. Softback. 152 pages. Write publisher for price information and further titles.

A Step-By-Step Guide To Personal Management for Blind Persons. American Foundation for the Blind, Inc., 15 West 16th Street, NY, NY 10011. 1970. Softback. 239 pages. Write for information.

Understanding "Senility" - A Layperson's Guide. Susan Thornton & Virginia Fraser. Revised Edition, 1982. Softback. 47 pages. Potentials Development. (See address above for more information.)

Why Salt the Peanuts? Sayings of the 5ᶜ Psychiatrist. Ben Weininger & Henry Rabin. Foreward by Charles Schultz. The Guild of Tutors Press, Los Angeles, CA. 1979. Softback. 127 pages. $3.95. (Excellent musings! —Editor.)

Aging Is a Lifelong Affair. Benjamin Weininger, MD & Eva L. Menkin. The Guild of Tutors Press. $3.95.

Work and Retirement. Stanley Parker. Allen & UNWIN, Inc., Winchester, MA. 1982. Cloth $28.50, Paper $9.95. 203 pages.